Monograph
Vertigo and Syncope

Balasubramanian Samivel MD DM
Professor
Institute of Neurology
Madras Medical College
Chennai, Tamil Nadu, India

Biju K Alexander MD
Consultant Neurologist
Marian Hospital Chapel
Kottayam, Kerala, India

Chandramouleeswaran Venkatraman MD DM
Former Professor
Institute of Neurology
Madras Medical College
Chennai, Tamil Nadu, India

Daniel Sweetson A MD DM
Consultant Neurologist
Government Mohan Kumaramangalam Medical College
Salem, Tamil Nadu, India

Deepa Avadhani MD DM
Assistant Professor
Department of Neurology
Sri Ramachandra Institute of Higher Education and Research
Chennai, Tamil Nadu, India

Deepti Ashok Kewalramani MD
Associate Consultant
Department of Neurology
Sri Ramachandra Institute of Higher Education and Research
Chennai, Tamil Nadu, India

Dulari Gupta MD DM
Associate Professor
Bharati Vidyapeeth Medical College
Pune, Maharashtra, India

Ganesh Vallampalli MD DM
Consultant Neurologist
Jayaditya Neuro Care
Kadapa, Andhra Pradesh, India

Gobinathan Shankar MD DM
Professor
Institute of Neurology
Madras Medical College
Chennai, Tamil Nadu, India

Guhan Ramamurthy MD DM
Consultant Neurologist
BG institute of Neurosciences
Tiruchendur, Tamil Nadu, India

Hemanth Kumar Arumugam MBBS
Clinical Research Fellow
Department of Neurology
Sri Ramachandra Institute of Higher Education and Research
Chennai, Tamil Nadu, India

Kavitha G Meikandan MD DM
Consultant
Department of Neurology
Ganesh Priya Hospital
Madurai, Tamil Nadu, India

Kranthi Karunakaran MD
Assistant Professor
Department of Pharmacology
Sri Ramachandra Medical College and Research Institute
Chennai, Tamil Nadu, India

Lenin S Palanisamy MD DM
Assistant Professor
Thanjavur Medical College
Thanjavur, Tamil Nadu, India

Mariappan V MD DM
Consultant Neurologist
Sri Jayam Medical Center
Cuddalore, Tamil Nadu, India

Mugundhan K MD DM
Senior Assistant Professor
Department of Neurology
Government Mohan Kumaramangalam Medical College Hospital
Salem, Tamil Nadu, India

Muthukumar Ramamurthy MS DLO Dip NB
Professor
Upgraded Institute of Otorhinolaryngology
Madras Medical College
Chennai, Tamil Nadu, India

Natuva Sai S Kumar DNB DM
Professor
Department of Neurology
Narayana Medical College
Nellore, Andhra Pradesh, India

Nelabhotla Sai Satya Saranya MD
Senior Resident
Institute of Neurology
Madras Medical College
Chennai, Tamil Nadu, India

Nirumal Khumar MD DM DrNB FEBN MRCP SCE(UK)
Assistant Professor
Saveetha Medical College and Research Institute
Chennai, Tamil Nadu, India

Noel James MD DM DrNB PDF Epilepsy FEBN FWHS SCE
Consultant Neurologist
Bensam Superspeciality Hospital
Nagercoil, Tamil Nadu, India

Philo Hazeena MD DM
Associate Professor
Department of Neurology
Sri Ramachandra Institute of Higher Education and Research
Chennai, Tamil Nadu, India

Prabaharan C MD DM
Consultant Neurologist
Neuro Foundation
Salem, Tamil Nadu, India

Prabaharan Umachandran MD DM
Assistant Professor
Government Viluppuram Medical College
Tamil Nadu, India

Prabash PR MD DM
Consultant Neurologist
SIMS Vadapalani
Chennai, Tamil Nadu, India

Ranjith Kumar Manokaran MD DM
Associate Professor
Department of Neurology
Sri Ramachandra Institute of Higher Education and Research
Chennai, Tamil Nadu, India

Sarala G MD DM
Professor
Institute of Neurology
Madras Medical College
Chennai, Tamil Nadu, India

Saranya Masilamani MD DM
Assistant Professor
PES Medical College
Kuppam, Tamil Nadu, India

Shaik Farheen Bhanu MD
Senior Resident
Department of Neurology
Sri Ramachandra Institute of Higher Education and Research
Chennai, Tamil Nadu, India

Sindhu Kalyanaraman MBBS
Consultant ENT Surgeon
Jhanvi ENT Clinic
Chennai, Tamil Nadu, India

Shrivarthan R MD DM
Consultant Neurologist, MGM Healthcare
Chennai, Tamil Nadu, India

Sudhir S Kothari MD DM
Head, Department of Neurology
Poona Hospital and Research Centre
Pune, Maharashtra, India

Sundar Shanmugam MD DM
Professor
Department of Neurology
Sri Ramachandra Institute of Higher Education and Research
Chennai, Tamil Nadu, India

Thamil Pavai N MD DM
Professor
Institute of Neurology
Madras Medical College
Chennai, Tamil Nadu, India

Venkata Sai Suhas Yadlapati
Senior Resident
Department of Neurology
Sri Ramachandra Institute of Higher Education and Research
Chennai, Tamil Nadu, India

Venkatesh Perumalsamy DM
Consultant, Department of Neurology
Velammal Medical College Hospital,
Athithi Neuro Clinic
Madurai, Tamil Nadu, India

Venkateswaran K Jeyaram MD DM
Assistant Professor
Madurai Medical College
Madurai Tamil Nadu, India

Venkatraman Karthikeayan MD DM
Consultant Neurologist
Kauvery Hospital
Chennai, Tamil Nadu, India

Vivek Mathew MD DM DNB
Professor
Department of Neurology
Christian Medical College
Vellore, Tamil Nadu, India

Foreword

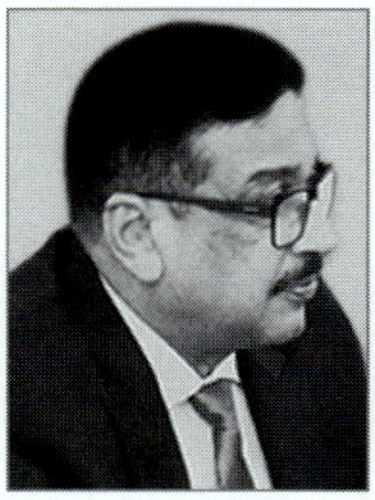

Mohan Kameswaran MS FRCS DSc
Director, Madras ENT Research Foundation, Chennai, Tamil Nadu
Awarded Padmashri and BC Roy Awards
Honorable Distinguished Professor, The Tamil Nadu Dr MGR Medical University, Chennai, Tamil Nadu, India
Chairman Emeritus, Indian Academy of Otorhinolaryngology and Head and Neck Surgery

It gives me great pleasure to write a foreword for the second edition of the book on "*Monograph*: *Vertigo and Syncope*", edited by Professor Lakshmi Narasimhan Ranganathan. Needless to say the book is a worthy successor to the first edition, which had a tremendous and enthusiastic reception. The book is a delicate balance between the "theory and practice", managing to give the readers a perspective of the intricate theoretical principles, which helps humans maintain their balance and sense of perception of their place in their environment while at the same time not sacrificing the importance of clinical practice. This is not so easily achieved in the field of vestibular medicine, but this book has managed to succeed in this endeavor where many previous iterations have failed.

The chapters on vertigo and balance are carefully curated and cover a gamut of topics both common and uncommon like the multimodal sensory integration of balance. The chapters on syncope are no less interesting and bring forth the multidisciplinary nature of the problem.

Overall, the book is an important and significant contribution to the science of vertigo and syncope and is a must read for students and practitioners in this field. I am sure the book will be of immense value to neurologists, neuro-otologists, otolaryngologists, internists, and family physicians. I have no hesitation in commending the book in the highest terms.

Foreword

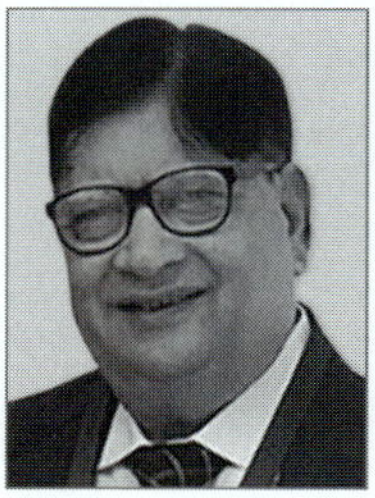

Kamalesh Tiwari MD FRCP
Dean, Indian College of Physicians (2025–2026)
Past President, Association of Physicians of India (2021–2022)
Former Professor and Head, Department of Medicine,
Sri Krishna Medical College and Hospital, Muzaffarpur, Bihar
Fellow of the Royal College of Physicians, Glasgow

As the Dean of Indian College of Physicians (ICP), I am pleased to recommend this second edition of the monograph "*Monograph*: *Vertigo and Syncope*", following the widespread acclaim for the earlier edition. The evaluation of vertigo and syncope continues to pose a diagnostic challenge across a range of clinical settings. These symptoms, though frequently encountered, are often complex in origin and require careful integration of clinical acumen with an understanding of underlying physiology. It is in this context, this book, edited by Professor Dr Lakshmi Narasimhan Ranganathan and team, assumes particular significance. This edition reflects a commendable effort to provide a comprehensive and structured approach to disorders of balance and transient loss of consciousness. The sections on vertigo are notable for their clarity and breadth, encompassing both common vestibular syndromes and more intricate aspects such as multisensory integration. The chapters addressing syncope are equally comprehensive, highlighting multifactorial etiology and the importance of a multidisciplinary diagnostic framework.

What sets this edition apart is its ability to present complex subject matter in a simple manner that is both accessible and academically rigorous. It offers practical guidance while remaining anchored in current scientific understanding—qualities that enhance its relevance to both trainees and experienced clinicians. This work will undoubtedly serve as a valuable reference for neurologists, otolaryngologists, internists, and general practitioners involved in the assessment and management of these symptoms. I commend Professor Narasimhan and the contributors for this significant and timely addition to clinical medicine.

Preface to the Second Edition

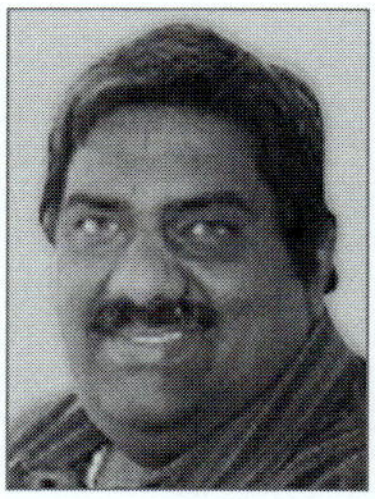

Lakshmi Narasimhan Ranganathan MD DM DNB(Internal Medicine) DNB(Neurology) FAAN FIAN FRCP(London and Glasgow) FACP PhD FEBN MNAMS
Professor and Head
Department of Neurology
Sri Ramachandra Institute of Higher Education and Research
Chennai, Tamil Nadu, India
Former Director and Professor, Institute of Neurology
Madras Medical College, Chennai, Tamil Nadu
President-Elect of Indian Academy of Neurology
President of World Headache Society
Adjunct Professor of IIT Madras, Chennai, Tamil Nadu
Adjunct Professor of Amrita Institute of Medical Sciences Kochi, Kerala, India

The human ability to maintain orientation and equilibrium, though often unnoticed in good health, is the result of an extraordinarily complex and finely tuned system. At the heart of this lies the vestibular apparatus—small in size, yet remarkable in function—an engineering marvel. Its disruption, however, can be both sudden and profoundly disabling, leading to distressing symptoms such as vertigo, imbalance, and even syncope. Disorders of balance and consciousness remain a diagnostic challenge due to their diverse etiologies and overlapping presentations. Vertigo alone accounts for a substantial proportion of outpatient consultations across multiple specialties, while syncope, often under-recognized, can stem from a wide range of cardiovascular, neurological, and systemic causes. For the clinician, deciphering these symptoms requires not only a firm grasp of anatomy and physiology but also a structured clinical approach. This second edition of "*Monograph: Vertigo and Syncope*" is an effort to equip practitioners with a comprehensive yet practical guide to these common but complex presentations. With updated content and reorganized chapters, it offers insights into vestibular structure and function, methods of clinical evaluation, central and peripheral vestibular disorders, and current management strategies.

Bringing this edition to life has been a collective endeavor. I express my sincere appreciation to all contributing authors for their scholarly input and clinical wisdom. I am especially grateful to Dr Arun Shivaraman, Dr Guhan Ramamurthy, Dr Srivarthan, and Dr Rithvik Ramesh and to my colleagues from Department of Neurology, SRIHER, for their committed involvement throughout this project. My thanks also go to Ms Asmi and Miss Sadhna for their diligent editorial support and to Jaypee Brothers Medical Publishers (P) Ltd, New Delhi, India, for their unwavering assistance in production.

Above all, I wish to thank my wife, Mrs Meera Lakshmi Narasimhan, and my daughter, Ms LN Mayura, for their constant encouragement and understanding. I remain deeply grateful to my parents, whose blessings continue to guide me.

Preface to the Second Edition

Preface to the First Edition

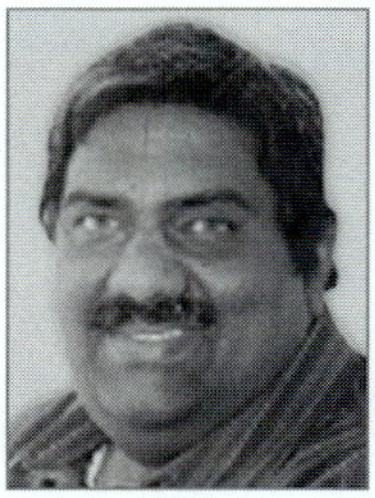

Lakshmi Narasimhan Ranganathan
MD DM DNB (Internal Medicine) DNB (Neurology)

The vestibular apparatus is deeply seated within the osseous inner ear. It plays a multivarious role from balance and equilibrium to gait and posture. The intricacies of the network connections are vastly complicated and functions to produce changes in the internal milieu, so as to produce adequate responses to maintain balance. Though the functioning of this small sized apparatus might not be noticed in the daily functioning of a healthy individual, its dysfunction can produce widespread ramifications. Due to the widespread connections, the symptoms can be severe and may be accompanied by autonomic manifestations causing the patient to seek a medical consultation immediately. Symptoms of vertigo constitute one-fifth of an outpatient department in general, neurology, and ear, nose, and throat practice. Syncope, a symptom that results from under perfusion of the brain can be multifactorial. It can be the presenting manifestation of various diseases. These symptoms can be a daunting task in the hands of an amateur to point at the diagnosis.

Hence it is essential on the part of the practitioner to have an extensive and in depth knowledge about these symptom manifestations. Akin to the multimodal vertical integration of vestibular cortex, this monograph aims to provide a vertical integration with an in-depth review on various aspects of vertigo including the anatomy and physiology of vestibular system, clinical examination and investigation of a vertiginous patient, diseases affecting central and peripheral vestibular networks, and medical and surgical management of the conditions. It also aims to provide an overview on approach to a patient presenting with syncope and brief descriptions about each cause.

I would like to thank the authors and coauthors for their immense contribution to the chapters. I would like to thank my registrars, Dr Arun Shivaraman and Dr Guhan Ramamurthy for their highest level of commitment and practical assistance in this project. I thank Ms Keerthana Vinodh for assisting me in this monograph. I would like to thank Ms Neha and team and Jaypee Brothers Medical Publishers (P) Ltd. for their support. Finally, I am indebted and grateful to my wife Mrs Meera Lakshmi Narasimhan and daughter Ms LN Mayura for their tolerance.

"I thank my mother Mrs Malathi Ranganathan for her blessing".

Contents

1 CHAPTER

Anatomical and Functional Correlates of Vertigo

Lakshmi Narasimhan Ranganathan, Shrivarthan R, Thamil Pavai N, Arun Shivaraman MM, Guhan Ramamurthy

ABSTRACT

The vestibular input is processed peripherally from the otolithic organs and semicircular canals. The macula of otolithic organs and crista ampullaris of semicircular canals provide information on the orientation of self to space. The information is transmitted to the vestibular nucleus, the processing of which is modulated by the cerebellum. The efferents from the vestibular nucleus through the medial longitudinal fasciculus and vestibulospinal pathway play a role in mediating reflexes that maintain gaze fixation and posture, respectively. The information provided is multimodally integrated with proprioceptive and visual information, forming the triangle of balance. The projections from the vestibular nucleus are transmitted to cortex through the thalamus. The vestibular information is integrated into the parietal, occipital, and temporal cortex, and thereby helps in deciphering space. Recent functional magnetic resonance imaging studies have localized the vestibular functions to the retroinsular cortex. The above-mentioned areas project through association fibers to the retroinsular cortex.

INTRODUCTION

The evolutionary process from quadrupeds to bipeds has resulted in centralization of weight toward the caudal end of body. This has been paralleled by the evolution in the intricacies of network processes that mediate balance. The balance is the net output produced by processing of information provided by vision, proprioception, and vestibular apparatus. The vestibular system deciphers the space around the person and helps maintain balance. The vestibular apparatus comprises separate organs for detecting linear and angular velocities. The nerve fibers arising from the receptors (hair cells) carry the impulses and relay in the brain, helping the individual to get oriented in space. Though the system is functionally contiguous and constitutes an intricate network from the periphery to the center, it can be arbitrarily divided into peripheral and central vestibular system.

PERIPHERAL VESTIBULAR SYSTEM

The entire vestibular apparatus is situated in the petrous temporal bone. The vestibular system contains the bony labyrinth that encloses the membranous labyrinth. Semicircular canals (SCCs) and otolith organs (utricle and saccule) form the membranous labyrinth. Bony labyrinth is filled by the perilymph, and membranous labyrinth is filled with the endolymph. The vestibule forms the central part of the membranous labyrinth into which the utricle, saccule, and (SCCs) open.

Semicircular canals detect angular velocity. Utricle and saccule (otolith organs) detect the linear velocity. The hair cells are the receptors that detect the movements in the organs and send impulses to the brain through vestibular component of 8th cranial nerve **(Fig. 1)**.

The perilymph, which fills the bony labyrinth, has chemical properties similar to extracellular fluid. Perilymph has high sodium concentration and low potassium levels. Endolymph behaves like intracellular fluid with high levels of potassium and low levels of sodium **(Fig. 2)**.

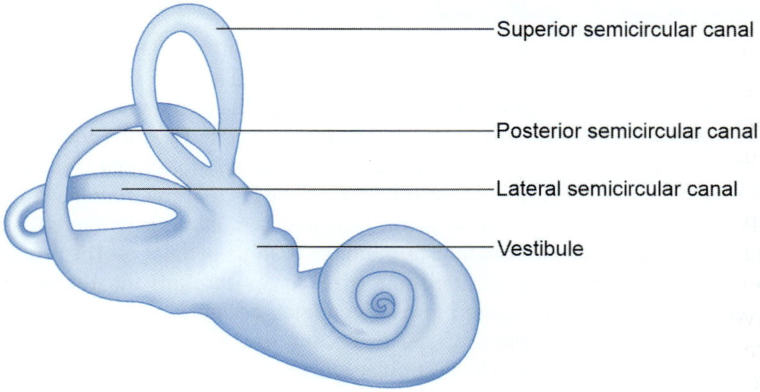

FIG. 1: Bony labyrinth containing semicircular canals and vestibule. The dilated ampulla of semicircular canals opens separately into the vestibule. The narrow ends of the superior and posterior semicircular canals open into the vestibule through a common opening. The narrow end of the lateral semicircular canal opens separately into the vestibule.

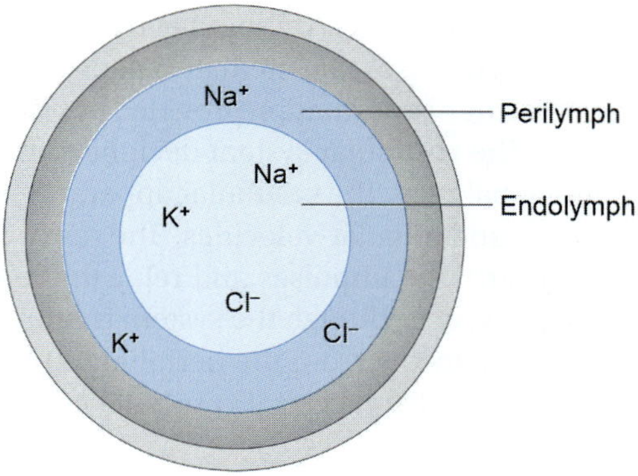

FIG. 2: Difference in the composition of perilymph and endolymph. Endolymph resembles intracellular fluid with high potassium and low sodium concentration. Perilymph resembles extracellular fluid with high sodium and low potassium concentration.

Planes

The movement of head occurs in three planes—(1) roll, (2) pitch, and (3) yaw.

- Roll axis (X-axis)—moving the head from one shoulder to another
- Pitch axis (Y-axis)—nodding the head, e.g., yes-yes movement
- Yaw axis (Z-axis)—nodding the head, e.g., no-no movement

Functional Anatomy of Rotational Movements

Semicircular canals detect the rotational movements of the head in relation to the environment. They are situated inside the bony labyrinth. There are three semicircular canals situated on each side, namely: (1) anterior/superior, (2) posterior, and (3) horizontal/lateral semicircular canals. They are oriented at right angles to each other. The orientation of the vertical (superior and posterior) canals is around 45° to the sagittal plane. The horizontal canal is oriented about 30° with that of the horizontal plane.

The SCCs open into the vestibule through five openings. Each SCC has a dilated end called ampulla, which opens into the vestibule. The narrow ends of the superior and posterior SCCs join together and form a common opening into the vestibule. Both narrow and dilated ends of the lateral SCC open separately into the vestibule. Each ampulla contains crista ampullaris, which is lined by the neuroepithelium. Hair cells and supporting cells arise from the neuroepithelium. The gelatinous structure, cupula, arises from the ridge of crista ampullaris and extends through the entire length of ampulla. The hair cells are covered by cupula.[1] The movement of the cupula causes movement in the hair cells, which creates the electrical impulses that are transmitted by the vestibular nerve **(Fig. 3)**.

In rotational movements of the head, there is also movement of fluid in SCCs. But, there is a lag in the movement of fluid in relation to head. The fluid moves toward the direction of ampulla in one side and away from ampulla on the other side. This relative motion deviates the cupula. This in turn causes movement in the hair cells, which is followed by depolarization and neurotransmitter release in the nerve fibers **(Fig. 4)**.[1]

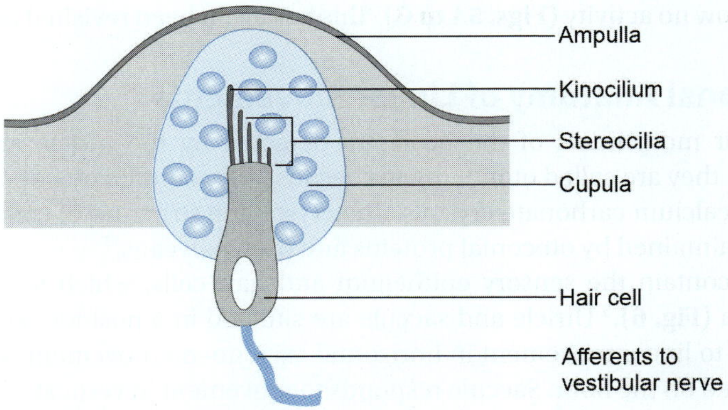

FIG. 3: Ampulla of semicircular canal containing a hair cell.

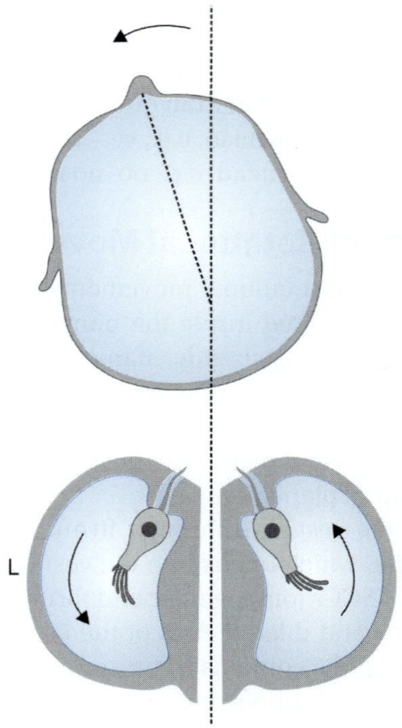

FIG. 4: On turning the head to the left side, differential movement of the endolymph that lags behind the head movement due to inertia causes deflection of the stereocilia and kinocilium of the hair cell. In the left ear (L), the deflection of the stereocilia occurs toward the kinocilium causing depolarization and increased firing. In the right ear (R), the deflection of the stereocilia occurs away from the kinocilium causing hyperpolarization and decreased firing.

The SCCs on both side form companions with each other—right anterior SCC and left posterior SCC, left anterior SCC and right posterior SCC, and right horizontal SCC and left horizontal SCC. This arrangement is called push-pull organization. If a person moves head to left side, the left horizontal SCC is depolarized and the right horizontal SCC is hyperpolarized. All the other four canals show no activity **(Figs. 5A to C)**. This has again been revisited in Chapter 8.

Functional Anatomy of Linear Movements

The linear movements of the head are detected by the utricle and saccule. Together, they are called otolith organs because they contain otoconia. Otoconia contains calcium carbonate crystals. The crystalline structure of calcium carbonate is maintained by otoconial proteins and proteoglycans.[2]

They contain the sensory epithelium and hair cells, which are embedded in macula **(Fig. 6)**.[3] Utricle and saccule are situated in a position so that utricle responds to linear movement in horizontal axis (no-no movement) as hair cells are situated on the floor. Saccule responds to movement in vertical axis[4] (yes-yes movement) as the hair cells are situated on the lateral wall **(Fig. 7)**.

As the head moves, the otolith organs also move, but there is a relative inertia in the movement of otolith organs because of the weight of the calcium carbonate

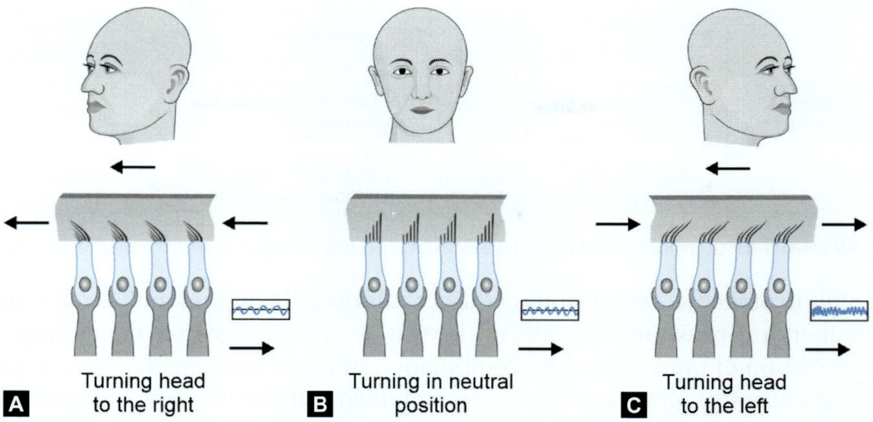

FIGS. 5A TO C: Ampulla of left semicircular canal in response to angular acceleration. (A) Movement of stereocilia away from kinocilia causing hyperpolarization of hair cell and a reduction in firing on turning the head to the right; (B) Equal degree of firing from hair cells of semicircular canals on either side while the head is in neutral position; and (C) Movement of the stereocilia toward the kinocilia causing depolarization of the hair cell and an increase in firing on turning the head to the left.

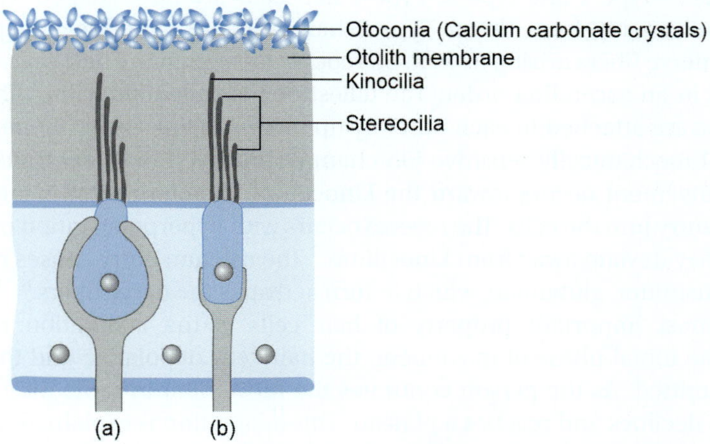

FIG. 6: Macula of otolithic organs containing type I (a) and type II (b) cells.

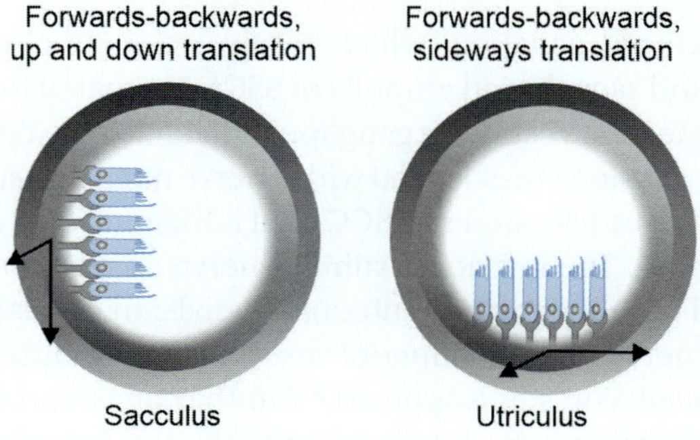

FIG. 7: Orientation of hair cells in the otolithic organs and the arrows showing translational motion in the corresponding direction.

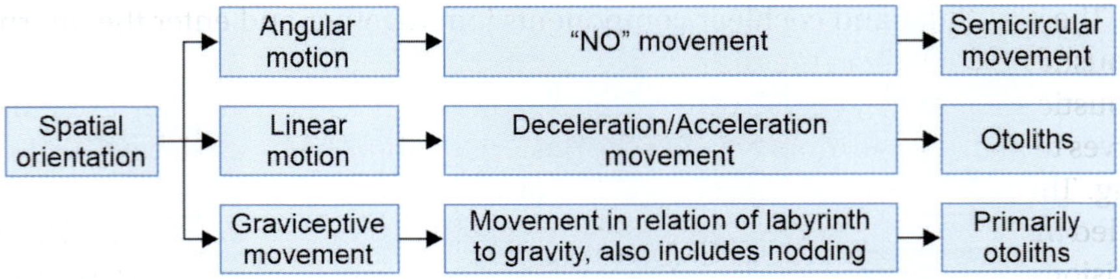

FLOWCHART 1: Components of spatial orientation and role of individual vestibular receptors.

crystals in otoconia. Dimensions of the crystals range between 1 and 50 microns.[5] This inertia causes the hair cells to depolarize or hyperpolarize depending on the direction of movement. The combination of linear and angular movements with graviceptive (gravity-related) perception contributes to spatial orientation, and the vestibular apparatus plays a crucial role in the perception of different components of spatial orientation **(Flowchart 1)**.[6]

Receptors (Hair Cells)

Hair cells are the primary receptor organs in vestibular system. They produce electrical signals that are transmitted by the vestibular nerve. There are two types of hair cells—type 1 and type 2. Type-1 hair cells are flask-shaped with single nerve fiber arising from them. Type-2 hair cells are cylindrical-shaped with multiple nerve fibers arising from it. Stereocilia arise from the hair cells. They are arranged in an ascending order. The tallest one is called kinocilia.[6] The tips of stereocilia are attached to each other by tip links. Tip links help in opening and closing of mechanically sensitive ion channels involved in signal transduction. As the movement occurs toward the kinocilium, depolarization is initiated by calcium entry into the cells. The reverse occurs with hyperpolarization of the hair cells as they deviate away from kinocilium.[7] The calcium entry causes release of neurotransmitter, glutamate, which in turn activates the nerve fibers.[6]

The most important property of hair cells is the adaptation response. During the initial phase of movement, the hair cells depolarize and the signals are transmitted. As the person continues the movement in same direction, the response declines and reaches a plateau. This adaptation is explained by gating-spring model for mechanoelectrical transduction.[8]

The Vestibular Ganglion and Nerve

The vestibular (Scarpa) ganglion, which receives the afferent fibers from the macula of utricle and saccule and ampulla of SSCs, is situated in the lateral part of internal auditory meatus. Vestibular ganglion is divided into superior and inferior divisions.[9,10] Each division is associated with a nerve fiber. The superior vestibular nerve arises from the utricle, superior SCC, and horizontal SCC and terminates in the superior ganglion. The inferior vestibular nerve arises from the saccule and posterior SCC and terminates in the inferior subdivision of vestibular ganglion.[9]

A small twig of nerve from the superior vestibular nerve ends in anterosuperior part of saccule called Voit's anastomosis.[9] Another anastomosis, the vestibulo-cochlear (Oort's) anastomosis, is formed between the inferior vestibular nerve and cochlear nerve.[9]

The vestibular and cochlear components join together and enter the internal acoustic meatus where they lie in a close relation with the facial nerve. The internal acoustic meatus is located within the petrous part of the temporal bone and serves to connect the inner ear with the posterior cranial fossa and is roughly 1 cm long. The medial end of the canal is *the porus acousticus* while the lateral end is called *the fundus*. The fundus is divided by a transverse crest into upper and lower divisions, and the upper division is further subdivided by a vertical crest (Bill's bar) into anterior and posterior compartments. In the meatus, the facial nerve is located in the anterosuperior portion of the canal, and the vestibulocochlear nerve occupies the posterior and inferior portions of the canal.[10] Vestibulocochlear nerve enters into the cranium after passing the internal acoustic meatus along the anterolateral aspect of the brainstem through cerebellopontine angle and enters the pons to terminate in the vestibular nuclear complex.[11]

CENTRAL VESTIBULAR SYSTEM

The central core of the vestibular system is forged by the vestibular nucleus, the cerebellar connections, and the extensive network of connections with extraocular muscles and extensor (cervical and truncal) musculature. The vast array of connections mediating vestibular reflexes help orient the body in space.

Vestibular Nuclear Complex

The vestibular nuclear complex consists of four major subgroups and several minor subgroups organized in the caudal pons and rostral medulla underneath the floor of the fourth ventricle. The major subgroups include medial, superior, lateral, and inferior nuclei.

The medial nucleus (Schwalbe nucleus) extends longitudinally as a medial column from the caudal pons to rostral medulla and is the longest vestibular nuclei. Medial vestibular nucleus receives afferent from the ipsilateral cristae of semicircular canals. Afferents from the macula of saccule and utricle also play a minor role. The medial nucleus projects through vestibulo-ocular projections to the extraocular muscles in mediating the VOR. It also projects through Deiters' tract to the medial rectus on the ipsilateral side. The medial vestibulospinal tract (MVST) receives contribution from the medial nucleus, travels in the ventral funiculus of the spinal cord, and influences the motor neurons of the cervical and upper thoracic spinal regions. The small neurons in the medial nucleus send commissural projections to the contralateral medial nucleus. The lateral nucleus (Deiters' nucleus) is lateral in the complex, and is separated from the medial nucleus by the dorsal acoustic striae. The lateral nucleus is functionally segmented into dorsal and ventral part. The ventral part receives afferent from the otolithic organs, and the dorsal part receives afferent from the vestibulocerebellum and the hemispheres of the cerebellum. The efferents from the lateral nucleus are carried in the lateral vestibulospinal tract (LVST), travel in the lateral funiculus of the spinal cord, and exert supranuclear control on the α-motor neurons throughout the entire spinal cord. The superior nucleus (Bechterew's nucleus) is confined to the caudal pons. It receives afferent from the cristae of semicircular canals. The efferents to the extraocular muscles arise from this nucleus and through medial longitudinal fasciculus mediate the VOR. It also sends output to the cerebellum and commissural projections to the contralateral side. The inferior nucleus (descending nucleus of Roller) is the inferior-most part of the vestibular nucleus. It receives afferent from vestibular end organs and cerebellum. The efferents project through the medial vestibulospinal tract to exert supranuclear control over anterior horn cells. The lateral and inferior vestibular nucleus send second-order neurons, projecting to the cerebellum the information from otolithic organs **(Fig. 8)**.

In addition to the four major nuclei, several groups of nuclei play a role in mediating the functions of vestibular system. These include group-Y nucleus, interstitial nucleus of vestibular nerve, group-L nucleus, group-F nucleus, group-X nucleus, and group-Z nucleus. Other groups of nuclei have also been described but their afferents and efferents have not been characterized and their role appears insignificant.[12-15]

Vestibular Network

The axons from cristae and macula stream through the brainstem to reach the vestibular nucleus. The fascicle containing the impulses from the semicircular canals bifurcates into ascending and descending rami. The ascending rami synapse in the superior nucleus and then continue to enter the cerebellum synapsing in the vestibulocerebellum (flocculonodular lobe). The descending ramus synapses in the medial vestibular nucleus. The second-order neurons travelling in the medial longitudinal fasciculus and ascending tract of Deiter, arising from the superior and medial vestibular nuclei, synapse in the extraocular muscles **(Table 1)**. The neurons from the medial vestibular nucleus also contribute to the MVST.[12,13]

The fascicle containing impulses from otolithic organ synapses in the inferior and lateral vestibular nucleus. The neurons arising from the lateral vestibular nucleus provide otolithic afferent to the cerebellum. Also, the second-order

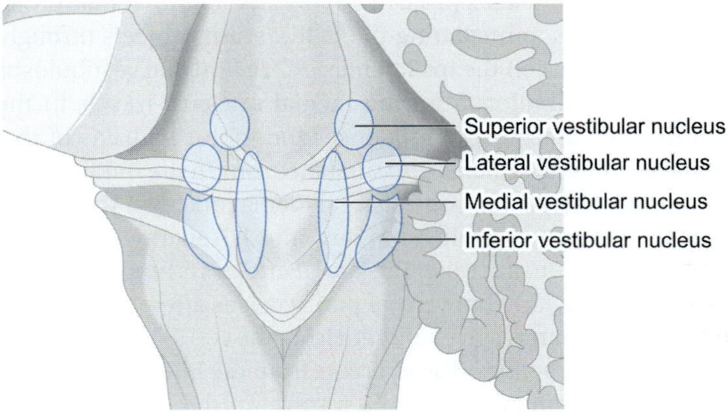

FIG. 8: The orientation of the major vestibular nuclear complex in the lower pons and superior medulla.

TABLE 1: Connections of individual semicircular canals (SCC) with the vestibular nucleus and the specific extraocular muscles activated.

Semicircular canal	Vestibular nucleus	Muscle activated	
		Ipsilateral	**Contralateral**
Anterior/Superior SCC	SVN, LVN, MVN	Superior rectus	Inferior oblique
Posterior SCC	LVN, MVN	Superior oblique	Inferior rectus
Horizontal/Lateral SCC	MVN	Medial rectus	Lateral rectus

(LVN: lateral vestibular nucleus; MVN: medial vestibular nucleus; SVN: superior vestibular nucleus)

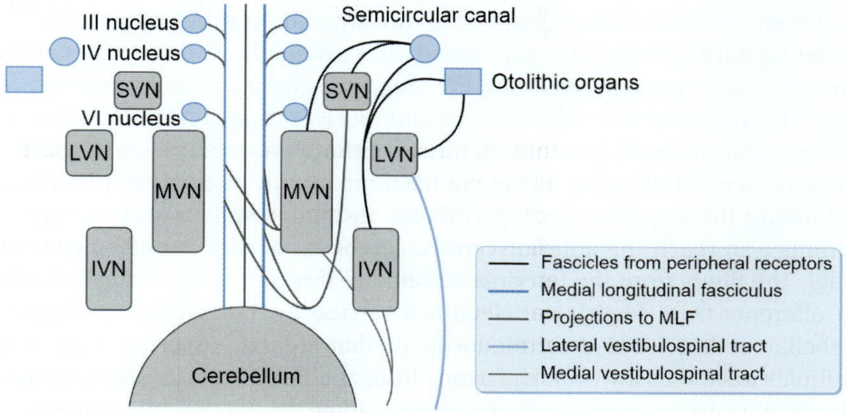

FIG. 9: Vestibular nucleus and extensive network of connections with afferents to and efferents from the nuclear complex.

(IVN: inferior vestibular nucleus; LVN: lateral vestibular nucleus; MVN: medial vestibular nucleus; SVN: superior vestibular nucleus)

neurons from the lateral nucleus form the lateral vestibulospinal reflex. The axons from the inferior vestibular nucleus form the MVST. The efferent nucleus located lateral to the abducent nucleus sends fibers that travel with efferent cochlear bundle to the peripheral vestibular system bilaterally.[16-18]

The inputs to the vestibular nucleus include cerebellar fibers that synapse in the dorsal portion of the lateral vestibular nucleus, inferior, medial, and superior vestibular nucleus. The commissural fibers project from the superior, medial, and inferior nucleus to the corresponding contralateral nuclei. These connecting fibers are predominated by projections from superior nucleus and are responsible for exerting inhibitory impulses. The activation of commissural projection by depolarization of a semicircular canal results in inhibitory impulses to the complementary canal on the contralateral side. This helps in potentiating the inhibition of the contralateral canal. This produces a differential coplanar activity. The commissural projections mediate the differential activity for the semicircular canals **(Fig. 9)**.[19]

Cerebellum: Role in Modulation

The cerebellum plays a role in modulating the function of vestibular nucleus and its connections. It also helps in integration of multimodal sensory input. The vestibular input forms a major afferent to the cerebellum that concerns spatial orientation. The primary vestibulocerebellar fibers contain fibers from the peripheral vestibular system that do not relay in the vestibular nucleus. It relays input from the semicircular canals to the ipsilateral vestibulocerebellum. The secondary vestibulocerebellar fibers contain fibers from otolithic organs that relay in the vestibular nucleus. The inferior and medial nuclei play a major role in the relay of information from the otolithic organs. The secondary fibers from the inferior and medial vestibular nucleus project to the cerebellum bilaterally. They contribute to the afferents of vestibulocerebellum bilaterally. They contribute to the afferent of the arc that plays a role in inflecting the vestibulospinal input.

The region of cerebellum concerned with orientation that receives afferent from vestibular nucleus includes the flocculus, paraflocculus, nodulus, and uvula. This region of cerebellum sends and receives reciprocal innervation from the vestibular nucleus. In addition, the oculomotor vermian region (lobules VI, VII) also receives afferent. These connections play a role in deciphering and modulating the impulses from peripheral vestibular system and in VOR. The afferents also reach the anterior vermis, cerebellar cortex, and deep cerebellar nuclei. The fibers from the Purkinje system are directed to the fastigial nucleus. The efferents from fastigial nucleus are carried in the inferior and superior cerebellar peduncles and terminate in medial, lateral, superior, and inferior vestibular nucleus. However, the axons from the Purkinje cells also send direct input to the vestibular nucleus. The efferent fibers to the vestibular nucleus are inhibitory to the vestibular nucleus **(Figs. 10 and 11)**.[20,21]

Reflexes

Vestibulo-ocular Reflex

The neural circuit that concerns the VOR produces ocular movement that is of equal amplitude in the direction opposite to the head movement. The

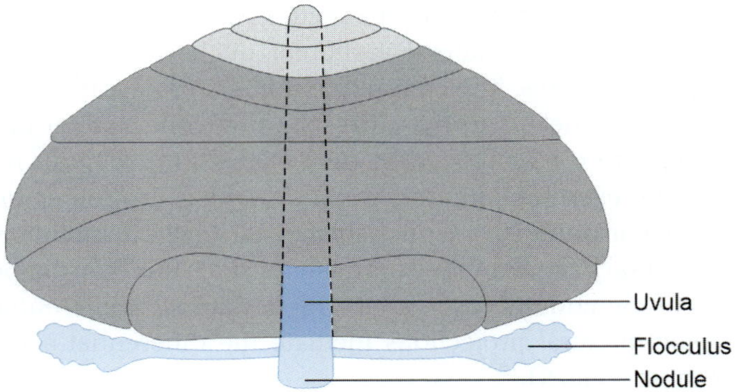

FIG. 10: Areas of cerebellum that primarily play a role in the modulation of vestibular information. These include flocculus, paraflocculus, uvula, and nodule of cerebellum.

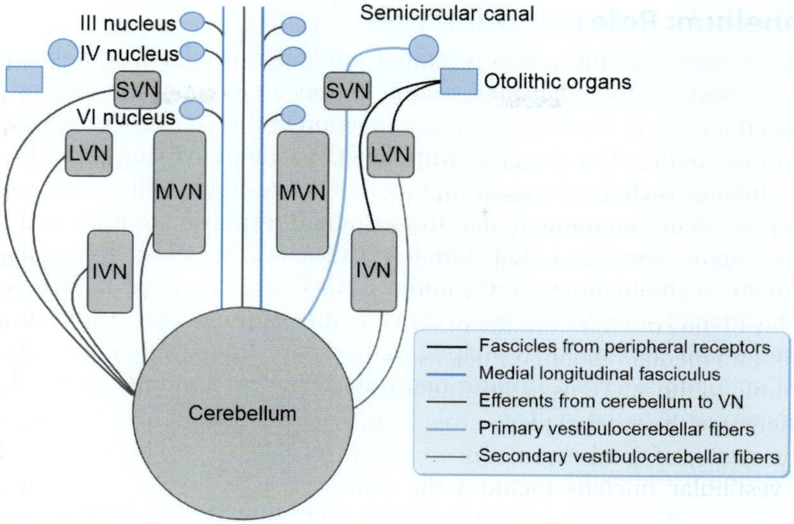

FIG. 11: Afferents to and efferents from the cerebellum. The primary vestibulocerebellar fibers do not rely in the superior vestibular nucleus. The secondary vestibulocerebellar fibers project bilaterally (not shown in this image)

(IVN: inferior vestibular nucleus; LVN: lateral vestibular nucleus; MVN: medial vestibular nucleus; SVN: superior vestibular nucleus; VN: vestibular nucleus)

information containing the change in spatial orientation from the cristae of the SCC is transmitted to the vestibular nucleus. The medial and superior vestibular nuclei are concerned with the reflex. These nuclei send projection to the nuclei concerning ocular movements **(Table 1)**. Efferents from these nuclei project to the yoked pairs in producing the opposite conjugate eye movement through the medial longitudinal fasciculus. The velocity of ocular movement produced in response to the angular movement of head is termed VOR gain. The VOR gain is a function of the angle of vergence. A larger VOR gain is required for objects closer to the subject as compared to distant objects for the same amplitude.

The VOR stabilizes gaze remarkably in response to head movements. The ocular movements lag by only 5 ms to the head movements in primate studies. The efficacy of VOR is such that the VOR gain produced is close to unity for angular velocity reaching 500° per second. VOR gain is close to unity.

$$\text{VOR gain} = \frac{\text{Change in the angle of the eye movement}}{\text{Change in the angle of the head movement}}$$

In voluntarily directing a gaze toward an object that is located beyond the visual field, it is essential for the ocular movements to be in the same direction as the head movement. VOR, which moves the eye in the direction opposite to the head, needs to be suppressed. The suppression of the vestibular nucleus is mediated by premotor saccadic and pursuit networks. These networks send a copy of the voluntary eye movement command that mediates the suppression of the vestibular nucleus. The VOR suppression is maximal at the early part of the voluntary eye movement and returns to normal values toward the end of the shift in gaze.[22,23]

Vestibulocollic Reflex

When the body of an individual is rotated suddenly with the head free to move, the head moves in the opposite direction to prevent its repositioning and helps in fixing the gaze on the target. The gaze fixation in this scenario is mediated by the vestibulocollic reflex. Together with the VOR, it helps in fixing gaze. The canal inputs mediate high-frequency component of the vestibulocollic reflex, whereas the low-frequency component and the sustained response are mediated by the otolithic inputs. The stimulation of the left SCC causes the head to turn to the right side. Bilateral stimulation of the anterior SCCs causes the head to turn upward with elevation of the chin. Similar to the VOR, the vestibulocollic reflex (VCR) also involves a well-developed trisynaptic pathway (vestibular afferents, vestibular nuclei, and cranial/cervical motor neurons).[24] The lag and latency in VCR are longer compared to the VOR.[24]

Vestibulospinal Reflex

The vestibulospinal reflex system is a highly efficacious and an intricate network of reflex system. It is fuelled by inputs from the peripheral vestibular system that is translated into dynamic stability and orientation of body in space mediated through skeletal muscles controlled by the vestibulospinal system. The gravity vector, which is a function of head position in space and linear acceleration, detected by the otolithic organs provides the input. The reflex system then produces the appropriate postural adjustments that are required to maintain balance. The vestibular system poorly differentiates lateral flexion of neck on body and lateral flexion of trunk. In either case, the otolithic organ on the ipsilateral side fires. The differentiation is produced by the afferents to this reflex system from propriospinal inputs and visual inputs that are required for finer deciphering of the orientation of body to space.[25]

The vestibulospinal reflex is mediated by lateral, medial, and caudal vestibulospinal tract. The LVST originates from the lateral vestibular nucleus. The fibers originating from the rostral and ventral portion of lateral vestibular nucleus terminate in the ipsilateral cervical segment of spinal cord and those from caudal and dorsal portion terminate in the lumbar segment of the spinal cord. These tracts increase the tone of the extensor muscles upon stimulation of the lateral vestibular nucleus. The afferents from otolithic organs to the ventral portion of the lateral vestibular nucleus are connected to the cell bodies of the LVST through interneurons. They also receive modulating input from the cerebellum. The MVST originates from the border between the medial and inferior, and inferior and lateral vestibular nuclei. They receive input from the semicircular canals and project to the cervical segment of spinal cord bilaterally. In contrast to the LVST, the medial tract receives monosynaptic afferent from peripheral vestibular system, projects bilaterally, is predominantly inhibitory, and receives inhibitory commissural projections from the contralateral medial vestibular nucleus. The caudal vestibulospinal tract originates from the medial and the descending vestibular nucleus and projects to the lumbar segment of the spinal cord. The functional significance is unknown. It is proposed that the part of nuclei that gives rise to the caudal vestibulospinal tract receives propriospinal input from the cervical region.[26,27] Experimental studies have shown that the impulses travelling through the vestibulospinal pathways are highly regulated and contain both excitatory and inhibitory signals. The ipsilateral excitatory signals travel through the LVST while the contralateral signals and ipsilateral inhibitory signals travel through the MVST.[24]

Cortical Processing

The vestibular nuclei receiving afferents from the peripheral vestibular system send projection to the contralateral thalamus. The ventral posterior complex of the thalamus receiving this information transmits it to the cortex. It merges with cortical areas responsible for other sensory modalities. It projects the information to parietal cortex (Brodmann area 3a, 2, and 5) responsible for somatosensory input. It also sends information to visual cortex, which plays a role in orienting visual field. The convergence of vestibular input into areas designated for vision and somatic sensation emphasizes the multimodal nature of processing. This is further reiterated by the presence of tracts that carry somatosensory information from proximal joints and muscles in close proximity to the vestibular tracts travelling from thalamus to cortex. The existence of a cortical area dedicated to vestibular processing has long been debated. However, recent functional magnetic resonance imaging studies have shown that the information from SCCs converge onto retroinsular cortex, parietal operculum, and posterior insula.[28-30] Based on experimental (animal) studies and human functional imaging modalities, a region of the cortex referred to as the parietoinsular vestibular cortex (PIVC) has been identified as the cortical centre for the vestibular system. The PIVC is also concerned with functions not typically associated with balance and vestibular functions like basic autonomic control, perceptual and motor decision-making, formation of mental imagery and mental rotation, higher level cortical processing concerned with spatial navigation, learning and memory, and representations of bodily self-consciousness.[31]

Sensory Integration for Spatial Orientation

The spatial orientation of self in space is a function established by integration of inputs from vestibular system, visual system, and proprioceptive stimulus. This is evident from multimodal processing at various levels. Though these systems establish balance, the functional modes operate through different receptors. This, in return, determines the frequency range of operations. The visual input operates at low frequency and vestibular input operates at high frequency. This is exemplified by the vection, a visual illusion in which the subject is tricked into believing that the self is in motion when large portions of visual fields are moving. An adjacent train that is starting to move provides the illusion that the subject is moving. This is because at such a low frequency, the stimulation of vestibular receptors is insufficient and is provided by visual stimulus. This is accepted by the cortex and indicates self-motion. On the other hand, when a train moves rapidly, the vestibular input suggests no motion, which is processed by the cortex. The contrast in frequency operation of the two systems is explained by the longer latency for visual input and different physical and biological properties of the peripheral receptor.

The integration of proprioceptive input is essential in fine interpretation of the orientation of the head and body. The differential interpretation between the lateral flexion of head on trunk and lateral flexion of the trunk is established by the added proprioceptive input to the vestibular processing. The integration is provided at the vestibular nucleus, cerebellum, and cortical levels. The dorsal aspect of lateral vestibular nucleus and caudal aspect of descending vestibular nucleus receive proprioceptive input. The anterior vermis of cerebellum receives vestibular input and proprioceptive input. This projects to the lateral vestibular nucleus and helps control the lateral vestibulospinal tract in mediating the vestibulospinal reflex. This multimodal sensory processing is essential for effective positioning of self in space. This also reduces the dependency on vestibular system for balance and helps in better adaptation when the vestibular apparatus dysfunctions. This principle also helps in the rehabilitation of a patient with vestibular dysfunction.[32]

CONCLUSION

The multimodal integration of the sensory input has helped in maintaining the erect posture of the bipeds. However, human studies are required to extrapolate information derived from animal studies to humans. With the advent of advanced neuroimaging, it is a practical possibility in delineating the networks and circuitry.

REFERENCES

1. Highstein SM, Holstein GR. The anatomical and physiological framework for vestibular prostheses. Anat Rec (Hoboken). 2012;295(11):2000-9.
2. Lundberg YW, Xu Y, Thiessen KD, Kramer KL. Mechanisms of otoconia and otolith development. Dev Dyn. 2015;244(3):239-53.
3. In: Purves D, Augustine GJ, Fitzpatrick D, Katz LC, LaMantia AS, McNamara JO, Williams SM (Eds). The otolith organs: The utricle and sacculus. Neuroscience, 2nd ed. Sunderland (MA): Sinauer Associates; 2001.
4. Jamali M, Sadeghi SG, Cullen KE. Response of vestibular nerve afferents innervating utricle and saccule during passive and active translations. J Neurophysiol. 2009;101(1):141-9.
5. Carlström D. A crystallographic study of vertebrate otoliths. Biol Bull. 1963;125(3):441-63.
6. Baloh RW, Kerber K, Honrubia V. Baloh and Honrubia's Clinical Neurophysiology of the Vestibular System, Vol 77. Oxford, UK: Oxford University Press; 2011.
7. Hudspeth AJ, Choe Y, Mehta AD, Martin P. Putting ion channels to work: Mechanoelectrical transduction, adaptation, and amplification by hair cells. Proc Natl Acad Sci USA. 2000;97(22):11765-72.
8. Hudspeth AJ, Gillespie PG. Pulling springs to tune transduction: Adaptation by hair cells. Neuron. 1994;12(1):1-9.
9. Lysakowski A, McCrea RA, Tomlinson RD. Anatomy of vestibular end organs and neural pathways. Otolaryngology Head and Neck Surgery, 3rd edition. St Louis, Missouri: Mosby; 1998. pp. 2561-84.
10. Rubinstein D, Sandberg EJ, Cajade-Law AG. Anatomy of the facial and vestibulocochlear nerves in the internal auditory canal. AJNR Am J Neuroradiol. 1996;17(6):1099-105.
11. Tascioglu AB. Brief review of vestibular system anatomy and its higher order projections. Neuroanatomy. 2005;4:24-7.

12. Gacek RR. Anatomy of the central vestibular system. In: Jackler RK, Brackmann DE (Eds). Neurotology, 2nd ed. Philadelphia: Mosby; 2005. pp. 75-90.
13. Brodal A, Pompeiano O. The vestibular nuclei in the cat. J Anat (Lond). 1957;91(4):438-54.
14. Gacek RR. Location of commissural neurons in the vestibular nuclei of the cat. Exp Neurol. 1978;59(3):479-91.
15. Gacek RR. Anatomical demonstration of the vestibulo-ocular projections in the cat. Acta Otolaryngol Suppl. 1971;293:1-63.
16. Pillsbury HC 3rd. Lorente de No's R. Anatomy of the eighth nerve. I. The central projection of the nerve endings of the internal ear; III. General plan of structure of the primary cochlear nuclei. Laryngoscope. 1933;43:1-38.
17. Lorente de Nó R. Vestibuloocular reflex arc. Arch Neurol Psychiat (Chic). 1933;30:245-91. DOI: 10.3233/VES-220034.
18. Gacek RR. The course and central termination of the first-order neurons supplying vestibular end organs in the cat. Acta Otolaryngol Suppl. 1969;254:1-66.
19. Ladpli R, Brodal A. Experimental studies of commissural and reticular formation projections from the vestibular nuclei in the cat. Brain Res. 1968;8(1):65-96.
20. Kotchabhakdi N, Walberg F. Cerebellar afferent projections from the vestibular nuclei in the cat: An experimental study with the method of retrograde axonal transport of horseradish peroxidase. Exp Brain Res. 1978;31:591-604.
21. Brodal A, Hoivik B. Site and mode of termination of primary vestibulocerebellar fibres in the cat. An experimental study with silver impregnation methods. Arch Ital Biol. 1964;102:1-21.
22. Della Santina CC, Cremer PD, Carey JP, Minor LB. The vestibulo-ocular reflex during self-generated head movements by human subjects with unilateral vestibular hypofunction: Improved gain, latency, and alignment provide evidence for preprogramming. Ann N Y Acad Sci. 2001;942:465-6.
23. Della Santina CC, Cremer PD, Carey JP, Minor LB. Comparison of head thrust test with head autorotation test reveals that the vestibulo-ocular reflex is enhanced during voluntary head movements. Arch Otolaryngol Head Neck Surg. 2002;128(9):1044-54.
24. Goldberg JM, Cullen KE. Vestibular control of the head: Possible functions of the vestibulocollic reflex. Exp Brain Res. 2011;210:331-45.
25. Roberts TDM. Neurophysiology of Postural Mechanisms, 2nd edition. London: Butterworth Publishers; 1978.
26. Schwarz DWF, Tomlinson RD. Physiology of the vestibular system. In: Jackler RK, Brackmann DE (Eds). Neurotology, 2nd edition. Philadelphia: Mosby; 2005. pp. 91-121.
27. Fredrickson JM, Kornhuber HH, Schwarz DWF. Cortical projections of the vestibular nerve. In: Kornhuber HH (Ed). Handbook of Sensory Physiology, VI/I, Vestibular System, Part I, Basic Mechanisms. New York: Springer Verlag; 1974.
28. Schwarz DWF, Fredrickson JM. The clinical significance of vestibular projection to the parietal lobe: A review. Can J Otolaryngol. 1974;3:381-92.
29. Reinis S, Landolt JP, Weiss DS, Money KE. Effects of deuterium oxide and galvanic vestibular stimulation on visual cortical cell function. J Neurophysiol. 1984;51(3):481-99.
30. Lopez C, Blanke O, Mast FW. The human vestibular cortex revealed by coordinate-based activation likelihood estimation meta-analysis. Neuroscience. 2012;212:159-79.
31. Frank SM, Greenlee MW. The parieto-insular vestibular cortex in humans: More than a single area? J Neurophysiol. 2018;120(3):1438-50.
32. Bronstein AM. Multisensory integration in balance control. Handb Clin Neurol. 2016;137:57-66.

2 CHAPTER

Insight into Multimodal Sensory Integration of Balance

Guhan Ramamurthy, Arun Shivaraman MM

ABSTRACT

Maintaining balance is a complex and dynamic process requiring the integration of sensory inputs from the vestibular, visual, and proprioceptive systems. These systems interact through multisensory integration to provide the brain with accurate information about body position and motion, enabling motor adjustments necessary for postural stability. This chapter explores the mechanisms of sensory integration for balance, emphasizing the role of neural pathways, reflexes, and cortical processes in processing sensory inputs.

Sensory reweighting, a dynamic adjustment of sensory contributions based on reliability and environmental conditions, is highlighted as a critical process for adapting to changes in sensory input or context. The chapter also examines the effects of sensory deficits, such as vestibular dysfunction, on balance control, demonstrating how impaired sensory integration can lead to instability. Experimental paradigms, including sensory withdrawal and perturbation methods, reveal insights into sensory weighting and its adaptation in maintaining balance. Additionally, the implications of multisensory integration for balance rehabilitation are discussed, with a focus on improving sensory processing and adaptive responses in individuals with balance disorders.

Understanding these processes offers valuable insights into designing effective interventions to reduce fall risks and enhance stability in diverse populations, including those with neurological impairments or age-related decline.

INTRODUCTION

Maintaining balance is a fundamental function of the human body, essential for performing everyday activities such as standing, walking, and running. The process of balancing, however, is not simple. It involves the continuous integration of sensory information from multiple sources, namely the *vestibular*, *visual*, and *proprioceptive* systems, which together provide the brain with the necessary data to adjust motor responses and maintain postural stability. These systems do not work independently; rather, they interact through a complex and dynamic process known as *multisensory integration*, which enables humans to adapt to constantly changing environmental conditions.[1]

The aim of this chapter is to delve into the intricate mechanisms by which multisensory integration occurs, the central role it plays in balance, and how impairments in this system can lead to balance disorders. By understanding the neuroanatomical, sensory, and motor processes that underpin balance control, we can better appreciate how the body maintains stability and how it can adapt to different contexts. We will also examine the impact of aging and various neurological conditions on this integration process and discuss potential rehabilitation approaches.

SENSORY SYSTEMS INVOLVED IN BALANCE CONTROL

Vestibular System

The vestibular system is one of the core sensory systems responsible for detecting head motion and spatial orientation. It is located in the inner ear and is composed of two major components: The semicircular canals and the otolith organs (utricle and saccule). The semicircular canals are responsible for detecting angular motion, or the rotational movements of the head, while the otolith organs detect linear acceleration and the position of the head relative to gravity.

When the head moves, the fluid (endolymph) within the semicircular canals shifts, stimulating hair cells located in the cupula. These hair cells convert mechanical motion into neural signals, which are transmitted to the vestibular nuclei (lateral, medial, superior, and inferior) in the brainstem through polysynaptic and disynaptic pathways. The otolith organs, on the other hand, contain small calcium carbonate crystals (otoconia) that shift in response to gravity, providing information about head tilt and linear acceleration.

The vestibular system plays a key role in stabilizing both posture and gaze. When the head moves, the vestibulo-ocular reflex (VOR) ensures that eye movements are adjusted to maintain stable vision. Simultaneously, the vestibulospinal reflexes control postural adjustments, ensuring that the body remains upright. These reflexes are fast and automatic, as the vestibular system constantly sends signals to the brain to regulate balance without the need for conscious thought.[2-4]

Visual System

The visual system contributes significantly to balance by providing the brain with information about the surrounding environment. Vision helps determine the position and motion of objects relative to the body and allows for depth perception, which is critical for navigating through space. Visual cues are particularly important in situations where proprioceptive or vestibular inputs may be compromised, such as when standing on unstable surfaces.

Information from the eyes is transmitted to the *visual cortex* in the occipital lobe, where it is processed and interpreted. Visual data is integrated with proprioceptive and vestibular inputs to create a coherent representation of the external environment. In terms of balance, visual cues provide feedback on the body's position relative to external reference points, such as the horizon or nearby objects.

The visual system also plays an essential role in anticipatory postural control, helping the brain to prepare for movements based on visual information. For example, when a person sees an obstacle in their path, the brain anticipates the need to adjust posture or change the walking pattern to avoid a fall. Additionally, the dorsal stream of visual processing, which links the visual cortex to the parietal cortex, helps coordinate movements based on spatial awareness.[4-6]

Proprioceptive System

Proprioception provides the brain with information about the position and movement of body parts. This system is composed of receptors located in the muscles, tendons, joints, and skin. Muscle spindles, e.g., detect changes in muscle length and the rate of stretch, while Golgi tendon organs monitor the tension in muscles and tendons. Joint receptors provide information about joint angles, and cutaneous receptors detect pressure and vibrations on the skin, particularly in the soles of the feet.

Proprioceptive inputs are vital for detecting subtle shifts in body position, especially when external visual or vestibular cues are limited. For instance, during quiet standing, the body makes constant microadjustments to maintain balance, largely driven by proprioceptive feedback from the feet, legs, and torso. This system is closely tied to reflex pathways in the spinal cord, such as the stretch reflex, which helps regulate muscle tone and adjust posture in response to changes in body position.

Proprioceptive information travels through the dorsal columns of the spinal cord to the somatosensory cortex, where it is integrated with other sensory inputs. This information allows the brain to monitor the relative position of body parts and make necessary adjustments to maintain balance. Loss of proprioception, as seen in conditions like peripheral neuropathy, can significantly impair a person's ability to maintain balance, especially when visual and vestibular cues are compromised.[1,4,7,8]

NEURAL INTEGRATION OF SENSORY INFORMATION FOR BALANCE

The process of maintaining balance involves the complex integration of sensory information from the vestibular, visual, and proprioceptive systems. This integration occurs across multiple levels of the nervous system, from the spinal cord and brainstem to higher cortical centers, including the cerebellum and parietal cortex.

Spinal Cord and Brainstem Integration

At the spinal cord level, proprioceptive feedback from muscle spindles, tendons, and joints is integrated with motor commands to produce reflexive adjustments in posture. These reflexes include the stretch reflex and Golgi tendon reflex, which help maintain muscle tone and regulate joint stiffness. For example, when the body sways slightly, proprioceptive inputs from the legs trigger adjustments in muscle activity to restore balance.[4]

The brainstem plays a pivotal role in integrating vestibular information with proprioceptive and visual inputs. The vestibular nuclei, located in the brainstem, act as a hub for processing signals from the vestibular apparatus. These nuclei also receive input from the cerebellum, which helps fine-tune motor responses. Together, these regions coordinate the reflexive adjustments that are necessary for maintaining an upright posture. These are mediated through medial and lateral vestibulospinal tracts. The medial vestibulospinal tract primarily from the medial vestibular nucleus travels in the medial longitudinal fasciculus and terminates in the cervical segment of the spinal cord, and hence, plays a role in the vestibulocollic reflex in modulating the postural alterations. The lateral vestibulospinal tract, primarily from the lateral vestibular nucleus travels in the anterolateral fasciculus and terminates in the rexed laminae VII and VIII. It modulates the neural activity necessary for mitigating postural displacements predominantly through extensor muscles.[9,10]

The reticular formation in the brainstem is involved in regulating muscle tone and postural reflexes. The lateral reticulospinal tract arises from nucleus reticularis gigantocellularis whereas, the medial reticulospinal tract arises from nucleus reticularis pontis, pars caudalis, and pars oralis. The reticulospinal tracts project from the reticular formation to the spinal cord, where they influence motor neurons that control the muscles involved in balance. This system is particularly important for anticipatory postural adjustments, stimulating or inhibiting the flexor or extensor muscles based on the task or posture.[11]

The Role of the Cerebellum and Inferior Olive

The *cerebellum* plays a crucial role in coordinating balance and fine-tuning motor control. It acts as a comparator, evaluating the difference between expected movements (based on motor commands–efferent copy) and actual sensory feedback (afferent copy). If there is a discrepancy, the cerebellum adjusts the motor output to correct the error. This process is essential for error correction in balance control and allows the body to maintain stability in dynamic environments through the cortico-ponto-cerebellar-thalamo-cortical loop by modulating the motor commands.

For example, when walking on an uneven surface, the cerebellum continuously monitors proprioceptive and vestibular inputs to detect any deviations from the expected movement pattern. If the body begins to sway or stumble, the cerebellum quickly adjusts muscle activity to restore balance.

Damage to the cerebellum, as seen in conditions such as ataxia, can result in significant balance impairments. Individuals with cerebellar damage often struggle with coordination, have difficulty maintaining posture, and are prone to falls. This highlights the critical role of the cerebellum in integrating sensory inputs and ensuring smooth, coordinated movements.[12]

The inferior olive serves as a hub for integration from motor cortex, spinal cord, trigeminal nucleus, vestibular nucleus, superior colliculus, and pretectum in its role for motor learning (error-based). It is mediated through the modulation of Purkinje cells and cerebellar nuclei.[13]

Higher Cortical Centers: Parietal Cortex and Beyond

While the spinal cord, brainstem, and cerebellum handle many of the automatic processes involved in balance, higher-order sensory integration and motor planning occur in the cerebral cortex. The parietal cortex is particularly important for processing spatial information and proprioceptive inputs, which contribute to an individual's awareness of their body position in space.

In addition to the parietal cortex, the premotor cortex, supplementary motor cortex, cingulate cortex, and primary motor cortex are involved in generating voluntary movements that are coordinated with balance control. These areas receive sensory input and use it to plan and execute movements that maintain stability, such as adjusting posture or preparing to step over an obstacle. These cortices are connected with mesencephalic locomotor regions, vestibular nuclei, pontomedullary reticular formations, and the intermediate zones of the spinal cord.[14,15]

MULTISENSORY INTEGRATION: INTRASENSORY VERSUS INTERSENSORY MECHANISMS

Intrasensory Integration

Intrasensory integration refers to the processing and integration of signals within a single sensory system. For example, in the vestibular system, inputs from the semicircular canals and otolith organs are combined to form a unified representation of head movement and orientation. The semicircular canals detect angular velocity, while the otolith organs sense linear acceleration and head tilt relative to gravity. Together, these inputs provide a comprehensive understanding of head motion, which is essential for maintaining balance.[16]

Intrasensory integration also occurs within the proprioceptive system, where inputs from muscle spindles, Golgi tendon organs, and joint receptors are combined to provide information about limb position and movement. This process allows the brain to accurately detect changes in body position and adjust motor commands accordingly.[17,18]

Intersensory Integration

Integrating sensory information from multiple systems provides key advantages, such as improving the accuracy and reliability of orientation and motion perception, ensuring redundancy to compensate for sensory impairments, and enabling flexible motor strategies to meet behavioral needs. This integration also helps to resolve sensory conflicts, e.g., distinguishing between self-motion and environmental motion, and combines inputs from different sensory systems (visual, vestibular, and proprioceptive) to generate body-in-space orientation.[19]

The variability across sensory systems arises from differences in their functional ranges. For example, the vestibular system's semicircular canals and otolith organs encode a broad range of head movements, supporting functions like the VOR during rapid movements. However, this wide range exceeds the smaller motion requirements for balance, resulting in a mismatch. In contrast, ankle proprioceptors are more specifically aligned with the range of motion necessary for standing balance.

Visual system variability depends on factors like contrast, spatial frequency, distance, viewing conditions (e.g., monocular or binocular), and cognitive processing. For example, visual motion detection is reduced in low-contrast or distant scenes. Motion detection thresholds further highlight these differences: Proprioceptive thresholds are the lowest, visual thresholds are slightly higher, and vestibular thresholds are significantly larger. These differences reflect the unique roles and limitations of each sensory system in balance and motion perception.[20]

Combining sensory inputs from multiple sources can effectively reduce overall variability, especially when multiple systems encode the same physical parameter. If all sensory systems exhibited similar levels of variability, a simple averaging approach might suffice. However, variability differences among sensory systems require a more sophisticated strategy. For instance, while vestibular inputs exhibit relatively high variability, excluding them entirely would not be optimal. This is because the vestibular system uniquely provides inertial motion-in-space information, which complements the relative motion cues derived from vision and proprioception. Excluding vestibular data could result in instability when visual or proprioceptive cues are unreliable.[21]

A maximum likelihood estimation model suggests that sensory inputs should be weighted based on their variability, with lower-variance signals contributing more to the overall estimate. This approach minimizes variability in the combined signal. However, in balance control, which functions as a closed-loop system, sensory signals interact dynamically. Noise from one sensory source can propagate through the system, affecting the variability of other sensory inputs. Over time, this interaction achieves a steady state of body sway, with the weighting of sensory inputs adapted to optimize specific goals, such as reducing sway displacement, velocity, or energy expenditure.[22]

SENSORY WEIGHTING AND REWEIGHTING: ADAPTING TO CHANGING CONDITIONS

The contribution of each sensory system to balance is not fixed; instead, the brain dynamically adjusts the relative importance, or weight, of sensory inputs depending on the situation. This process is known as sensory reweighting and allows the brain to adapt to changing environmental conditions or sensory deficits.

Environmental Influences on Sensory Reweighting

The environment plays a significant role in determining which sensory inputs are most reliable for balance control. For example, in well-lit conditions with stable surfaces, the brain may rely more on visual inputs to maintain balance. However, in low-visibility conditions, such as walking at night, visual inputs become less reliable, and the brain increases its reliance on proprioceptive and vestibular feedback.

Similarly, when walking on a compliant or unstable surface, such as sand or a foam cushion, proprioceptive feedback from the feet may be less reliable, leading the brain to prioritize visual and vestibular information. This ability to reweight sensory inputs based on environmental conditions is critical for maintaining balance in a wide range of situations.[18]

Experimental Approaches to Balance Control

Researchers use two main paradigms to investigate sensory contributions to balance:

1. *Sensory withdrawal and distortion*: In these experiments, specific sensory inputs are either removed or distorted to evaluate their role in balance. For example, closing the eyes eliminates visual input, leading to increased sway, while standing on a compliant surface disrupts proprioception, further destabilizing posture. These changes reveal how vision and proprioception are critical for maintaining stability. When both are impaired, reliance shifts to the vestibular system, which is less effective due to its inherently higher variability.
2. *Perturbation methods*: Here, targeted stimuli are used to challenge specific sensory systems and assess the resulting balance responses. For instance, moving visual scenes or tilting surfaces elicit sway responses that highlight the contributions of vision and proprioception, respectively. These experiments also help determine the relative importance—or "weights"—of different sensory inputs in maintaining balance under varying conditions.[18,23]

Sensory Weighting and Adaptation

Sensory inputs are integrated through a weighted system, where the contribution of each sensory modality depends on its reliability. Noisier systems, such as the vestibular system, are assigned lower weights compared to more stable inputs like proprioception. This dynamic process, known as sensory reweighting, allows the nervous system to adjust to environmental changes or sensory impairments.

For instance, during experiments with surface tilt stimuli, individuals with normal sensory function adapt their reliance on proprioception and vision based on the amplitude of the stimulus. In contrast, individuals with vestibular loss cannot adjust their sensory weights as effectively, leading to reduced balance control in challenging conditions.[18,24]

Challenges during Sensory Transitions

Sudden changes in sensory inputs, such as stepping onto a compliant surface or experiencing visual distortion, can temporarily destabilize balance. While the nervous system reweights sensory inputs to restore stability, this process takes time, leaving individuals vulnerable to instability during the transition. For example, after standing on a sway-referenced surface, where proprioceptive input is minimized, transitioning back to firm ground can result in transient oscillatory body sway. This instability arises from the delayed recalibration of sensory weights.[18]

IMPLICATIONS FOR BALANCE DISORDERS AND REHABILITATION

Understanding the dynamic integration of sensory inputs provides valuable insights into balance control, especially in individuals with sensory or neurological impairments. For instance, those with bilateral vestibular loss rely entirely on proprioception in the absence of visual input, as they cannot reweight sensory contributions effectively. Similarly, individuals with unilateral vestibular loss show increased reliance on proprioception to compensate for the variability in vestibular signals.

Experimental findings also highlight the importance of feedback mechanisms in balance control, where sensory inputs and motor responses interact to maintain stability. Advanced modeling approaches that incorporate sensory weights, time delays, and neural control parameters have proven effective in explaining balance behaviors. These models can also guide the development of targeted rehabilitation strategies for individuals with balance disorders.

CONCLUSION

Multisensory integration is the cornerstone of balance control, allowing the body to maintain stability in a wide range of environments and situations. The integration of sensory inputs from the vestibular, visual, and proprioceptive systems provides the brain with a comprehensive understanding of body position and motion, enabling rapid and precise motor adjustments.

Through dynamic processes such as sensory reweighting, the brain can adapt to changing environmental conditions and sensory deficits, ensuring that balance is maintained even when one sensory system is compromised. However, when sensory integration is impaired, whether due to aging, injury, or neurological disease, balance control can be severely disrupted, leading to instability and an increased risk of falls.

Understanding the mechanisms of multisensory integration provides valuable insights into the development of effective rehabilitation strategies for individuals with balance disorders. By challenging the sensory systems and improving the brain's ability to integrate and reweight sensory inputs, rehabilitation programs can help individuals improve their balance, reduce their risk of falls, and enhance their overall quality of life.

REFERENCES

1. Bronstein AM. Multisensory integration in balance control. Handb Clin Neurol. 2016;137: 57-66.
2. Mathews MA, Camp AJ, Murray AJ. Reviewing the role of the efferent vestibular system in motor and vestibular circuits. Front Physiol. 2017;8:1-15.
3. McCall AA, Miller DM, Yates BJ. Descending influences on vestibulospinal and vestibulosympathetic reflexes. Front Neurol. 2017;8:112.
4. MacKinnon CD. Sensorimotor anatomy of gait, balance, and falls. Handb Clin Neurol. 2018;159:3-26.

5. Drew T, Marigold DS. Taking the next step: Cortical contributions to the control of locomotion. Curr Opin Neurobiol. 2015;33:25-33.
6. Bronstein AM, Guerraz M. Visual-vestibular control of posture and gait: Physiological mechanisms and disorders. Curr Opin Neurol. 1999;12(1):5-11.
7. Mileusnic MP, Brown IE, Lan N, Loeb GE. Mathematical models of proprioceptors. I. Control and transduction in the muscle spindle. J Neurophysiol. 2006;96(4):1772-88.
8. Mildren RL, Strzalkowski ND, Bent LR. Foot sole skin vibration perceptual thresholds are elevated in a standing posture compared to sitting. Gait Posture. 2016;43:87-92.
9. Carpenter MB. Core text of neuroanatomy, 4th edition. Baltimore: Williams & Wilkins; 1991.
10. Abzug C, Peterson BW. Antidromic stimulation in the ponto-medullary reticular formation of local axon branches of contralateral vestibular neurons. Brain Res. 1973;64:407-13.
11. Schepens B, Drew T. Independent and convergent signals from the pontomedullary reticular formation contribute to the control of posture and movement during reaching in the cat. J Neurophysiol. 2004;92:2217-38.
12. Thach WT. Timing of activity in cerebellar dentate nucleus and cerebral motor cortex during prompt volitional movement. Brain Res. 1975;88:233-41.
13. Lang EJ, Apps R, Bengtsson F, Cerminara NL, De Zeeuw CI, Ebner TJ, et al. The roles of the olivocerebellar pathway in motor learning and motor control. A consensus paper. Cerebellum. 2017;16:230-52.
14. Lemon RN. The G. L. Brown Prize Lecture. Cortical control of the primate hand. Exp Physiol. 1993;78(3):263-301.
15. Fukushima K. Corticovestibular interactions: Anatomy, electrophysiology, and functional considerations. Exp Brain Res. 1997;117(1):1-16.
16. Merfeld DM. Signal detection theory and vestibular thresholds: I. Basic theory and practical considerations. Exp Brain Res. 2011;210(3-4):389-405.
17. Bosco G, Poppele RE. Broad directional tuning in spinal projections to the cerebellum. J Neurophysiol. 1993;70:863-6.
18. Peterka RJ. Sensory integration for human balance control. Hand Clin Neurol. 2018;159: 27-42
19. Mergner T, Rosemeier T. Interaction of vestibular, somatosensory and visual signals for postural control and motion perception under terrestrial and microgravity conditions–a conceptual model. Brain Res Rev. 1998;28:118-35.
20. Fitzpatrick R, McCloskey DI. Proprioceptive, visual and vestibular thresholds for the perception of sway during standing in humans. J Physiol (Lond). 1994;478(Pt 1):173-86.
21. Ernst MO, Banks MS. Humans integrate visual and haptic information in a statistically optimal fashion. Nature. 2002;415:429-33.
22. Van der Kooij H, Peterka RJ. Non-linear stimulus–response behavior of the human stance control system is predicted by optimization of a system with sensory and motor noise. J Comput Neurosci. 2011;30:759-78.
23. Jeka J, Oie KS, Kiemel T. Multisensory information for human postural control: Integrating touch and vision. Exp Brain Res. 2000;134:107-25.
24. Asslander L, Peterka RJ. Sensory reweighting dynamics following removal and addition of visual and proprioceptive cues. J Neurophysiol. 2016;116:272-85.

3

CHAPTER

Clinical Examination and Evidence-based Approach to Vertigo

Sudhir S Kothari, Venkatraman Karthikeayan, Venkateswaran K Jeyaram

ABSTRACT

Dizziness is a common symptom that a physician encounters in day-to-day practice. Like in most areas of neurology, the approach to a dizzy patient is a four-step process: History-hypothesis-examination-investigation. History focuses on understanding, clarifying, and defining the patient's complaint and trying to categorize it into one of the following categories, namely true vertigo, presyncope, disorders of balance, or psychogenic. The examination includes general medical, neurological, and neuro-otological examinations and is aimed at trying to confirm and then further narrow down the diagnostic hypothesis, into central or peripheral causes of vertigo, and then the further subtypes, e.g., different varieties of benign paroxysmal positional vertigo.

The assessment of eyes and eye movements forms a major part of the neuro-otological examination, including assessment of eye movements, nystagmus, the head impulse test, etc.

When a patient presents to the emergency department with acute onset dizziness, we can use what is called the TiTrATE (timing, triggers, and targeted examination) approach, in order to not miss potentially dangerous causes like stroke.

INTRODUCTION

Dizziness is one of the most common complaints in medicine. It contributes to about 30% of cases in the general population.[1] A majority of these patients have multiple consultations in vain due to the lack of methodological approach. When faced with a dizzy patient, the physician counters the problem of understanding the symptom. The word dizzy is often used by the patient to describe a number of symptoms such as vertigo, syncope, presyncope, gait instability, generalized weakness, and anxiety. When a patient presents with dizziness, it is imperative to define what he exactly means, when he says dizzy. This is achieved by a patterned approach.

The road map to the diagnosis is as follows:

History → Hypothesis → Examination → Investigation

So, essentially the history helps create some working hypothesis, which is further supported by examination, and investigations must be used mainly to confirm the hypothesis or else rule it out and encourage another hypothesis. Any short-cut method away from this approach will lead to unwanted investigations that burden the patient's economy and end up in losing the patients trust in the treating physician.

Acute presentation of dizziness needs a different approach since they may have a brainstem or cerebellar stroke as the cause and so, there is a sense of urgency.

DEFINITIONS

Let us begin by reviewing the international consensus definitions for major vestibular symptoms.

Dizziness is the sensation of disturbed or impaired spatial orientation without a false or distorted sense of motion. This includes sensations sometimes referred to as giddiness, lightheadedness, or nonspecific dizziness but does not include a vertigo.

Presyncope is the sensation of impending loss of consciousness. This sensation may or may not be followed by syncope. When patient reports lightheadedness, it should be as presyncope, dizziness, or both.

Syncope is transient loss of consciousness due to transient global cerebral hypoperfusion characterized by rapid onset, short duration, and spontaneous complete recovery.

Vertigo is the sensation of self-motion (of head/body) when no self-motion is occurring or the sensation of distorted self-motion during an otherwise normal head movement.

Unsteadiness is the feeling of being unstable while seated, standing, or walking without a particular directional preference.

Acute vestibular syndrome defined by rapid onset of vertigo, nausea or vomiting, unsteadiness with head motion intolerance, and nystagmus lasting for days-to-weeks. The symptoms develop in seconds to hours. These are usually self-limited and mostly presumed viral etiology. The differential diagnosis includes vestibular neuritis, multiple sclerosis, drug intoxication and posterior fossa tumors, infarction, and hemorrhage.

HISTORY

History taking is the first and the most important step on the road to diagnosis. The focused history leads to a postulated structural and etiological hypothesis pointing to a directed examination and a targeted investigation.

From the history one should try and categorize patients into one of the following:

- Vertigo
- Presyncope
- Unsteadiness or disequilibrium
- Psychogenic

Vertigo

If the patient describes his/her symptoms as a clear spinning or rotatory or whirling sensation, it is more in favor of a vertigo. Aggravation of the symptom by head movements, such as looking up or down, turning to one side, rolling over in the bed, lying down in the bed, or getting up from the bed, makes the diagnosis of vertigo more likely. Some patients describe the feeling as swaying in the boat or being pushed to one side. Some may even describe it as being thrown backward.

It is a big step, if we narrow down the diagnosis to vertigo, since that points the problem to the vestibular apparatus, either peripheral or its central connections. There are caveats though in this "quality" based approach to dizziness. Sometimes, patients may not be able to describe their symptom properly even though it is "true vertigo", e.g., due to benign paroxysmal positional vertigo (BPPV). They may just call it a heaviness or numbness in their head lasting for a few seconds, when they turn in bed. The clue here is the trigger and the timing. So, we use all three points for diagnosis—quality of dizziness, timing, and triggers. Using only one, e.g., just description of the dizziness or "quality" is liable to lead to diagnostic errors.

Once we have diagnosed it as true vertigo, the next step would be to differentiate the various causes of vertigo. This is done by distinguishing the peripheral from the central vertigo and also by the duration of individual episodes of vertigo **(Tables 1 and 2)**.[2]

TABLE 1: Causes of true vertigo according to duration of spells.

Few seconds	*Peripheral cause*: Unilateral loss of vestibular function, late stages of acute vestibular neuronitis, late stages if Ménière's disease
Several seconds to minutes	Benign paroxysmal positional vertigo, perilymphatic fistula
Several minutes to 1 hour	Posterior transient ischemic attack, perilymphatic fistula
Hours	Ménière's disease, stroke, migraine, acoustic neuroma, perilymphatic fistula
Days	Vestibular neuritis, stroke, migraine, multiple sclerosis
Continuous	Usually psychogenic (constant vertigo lasting for weeks without improvement)

Note: Migraine and psychogenic can cause any of the above.

TABLE 2: Differences between central and peripheral vertigo.

Features	Central vertigo	Peripheral vertigo
Illness	May appear deceptively mild	Patient may look very ill
Ataxia	More	Less
Feeling of vertigo	May be less	May be more
Tinnitus or deafness	Usually absent (except in anterior inferior cerebellar artery ischemia)	May be present (not always)
Brainstem symptoms/signs diplopia, dysarthria, dysphagia, dysphonia, paresthesia, etc.	May be present (but not always)	Absent

Differentiating a central and peripheral vertigo is usually easily possible from the history and examination.[2]

Peripheral vertigo is more distressing and most commonly associated with ear fullness, unsteadiness tinnitus, or hearing loss. The severity of the vertigo, nausea, and vomiting are usually concordance in peripheral vertigo. Peripheral vertigo cannot have the so called "Ds".

On the contrary, central vertigo may be mild and discordant to their severity. They will be accompanied by brainstem symptoms such as diplopia, dysarthria, dysphagia, dysphonia, dysesthesia, weakness, or limb ataxia. If the patient has vomiting or ataxia discordant to the subjective feeling of vertigo, central cause should be suspected. If the vertigo is accompanied by headache, the differentials should be either a central vertigo or a brainstem migraine. An associated neck pain should lead the search for vertebral artery dissection or again migraine.

Central vertigo can be deceptively benign looking, but can be dangerous if missed.

Presyncope

Syncope is associated with a transient loss of consciousness and, therefore, is easy to differentiate from dizziness and vertigo. Presyncope is characterized by a feeling that he or she might pass out. It may also be associated with darkening of vision. This is due to reduced blood flow to the brain. The most common cause is vasovagal or hypovolemia, but it may be due to cardiac disorders, such as arrhythmias, valvular heart diseases, or due to ischemic cardiac diseases. Postural hypotension occurs due to intravascular volume loss, autonomic dysfunction due to conditions, like diabetes, is an important cause. If it is precipitated by stress, pain, emotion, and cough, micturition vasovagal syncope should be considered. Presyncope occurs only on assuming an erect posture suddenly from a supine position or while standing for long time. It never occurs while lying in the bed or rolling side to side in the bed **(Table 3)**. One can easily check for postural hypotension by measuring the standing and supine blood pressure.

Unsteadiness or Disequilibrium

Imbalance or unsteadiness or disequilibrium is basically a feeling of loss of balance or feeling of unsteadiness. This would happen only when one is walking or getting up. It will be aggravated by walking on uneven ground or turning in the dark. The patient does not feel true spinning or rotatory sensation. This sensation reduces when another sensory modality comes to aid like vision or touch. The causes of imbalance are myriad and clinical clues and a full neurological examination,

TABLE 3: Dizziness: Common triggers.

On lying down or turning in bed	True vertigo
On getting up suddenly from sitting position	Faintness (check standing blood pressure)
Walking or turning	Loss of balance
When stressed or overworked	Psychogenic

TABLE 4: Causes of loss of balance or unsteadiness.		
Localization	**Disorders**	**Clues**
Cerebral	Binswanger's disease, isolated gait apraxia	Mental change, dysarthria, urgency, shuffling gait
Basal ganglia	Parkinsonism	Hypokinesia, rigidity, tremor, reduced arm swing
Cerebellum	Cerebellar ataxia	Broad based gait, limb ataxia, dysarthria, eye signs
Spinal cord	Myelopathies	Spasticity, brisk reflexes, up going plantars, impaired position, and vibration at toes
Peripheral nerve	Neuropathies	Absent deep tendon jerks, impaired sensations
Vestibular	Bilateral vestibulopathy	Oscillopsia, only gait ataxia, head impulse positive bilaterally

with a focus on the gait can help in differentiating the causes **(Table 4)**. Such patients may say they are feeling dizzy, but in actual fact they have either a problem leading to imbalance, ranging from Binswanger's disease, cerebellar ataxia, Parkinson's disease, or a spondylotic myelopathy to sensory ataxia due to B12 deficiency or diabetic neuropathy. They need proper neurological evaluation and treatment. Such patients will probably feel even worse when treated with the routine "vestibular suppressant" drug therapy.

Psychogenic

Patients can feel dizzy when under excessive stress, anxiety, depression, or feelings of insecurity. It may be described as lightheadedness or heavy head, tingling and numbness in the head, or instability to think clearly. There is often a clear relation to the psychological stressor and there is usually no relation to posture or change of position.

After getting a hypothesis by "slotting" the patient into one of these four categories, one must also consider timing and triggers to see if the category is appropriate. For example, if the patient has a clear sensation of rotation but it only happens when he stands up, one should check for postural hypotension. Similarly, even if the patient says he feels lightheaded but it is only for a few seconds and on looking up, one should check for BPPV.

In addition, we must keep in mind that patients can have more than one type of dizziness especially elderly patients. For example, psychogenic dizziness may be triggered by anxiety after an initial attack of BPPV or even micturition syncope. So one should focus on the first attack and also ask about each episode of dizziness separately and understand them individually before labeling the patient under one banner. A thorough medication history especially for aminoglycosides, diuretics, antidepressants, alcohol, and antipsychotics should be asked to rule out the drug induced causes of dizziness.

Common etiologies that are associated with each category are summarized in **Table 5**. Summary of the characteristics of each group is given in **Box 1**.

TABLE 5: Common causes.

True vertigo				
Peripheral	**Central**	**Presyncope**	**Loss of balance**	**Psychogenic**
• Benign paroxysmal positional vertigo • Vestibular neuritis • Ménière's disease	• Migraine • Stroke • Demyelination/ tumor	• Postural hypotension • Vasovagal attacks • Hyperventilation • Low cardiac output states	• Various neurological causes ○ Binswanger's ○ Parkinson's ○ Cerebellar ○ Myelopathy ○ Neuropathy ○ Bilateral vestibular failure, e.g., ototoxicity	• Stress • Anxiety • Depression • Watch out for mild forms of type 1–3, or poor descriptions by anxious patients

BOX 1 Summary of the characteristics of each group.

Dizziness type 1 or true vertigo:
- Essentially vestibular
- Spinning or definite rotation
- Precipitated by fast head movement
- Getting up/lying down
- Even turning in bed

Dizziness type 2 or presyncope:
- Essentially cardiovascular
- Faintness or darkness
- When upright or on getting up

Dizziness type 3 or loss of balance:
- Basically unsteadiness
- Feeling of imbalance
- When standing or walking
- Not when sitting or in bed
- Increased by uneven ground or turning

Dizziness type 4 or psychogenic:
- Vague
- Numbness in head
- Heavy or light headedness
- Unable to think clearly
- Some abnormal head sensation, not fitting in type 1–3

EXAMINATION

Physical examination in vestibular disorders play a major role in confirming the hypothesis put forth after history. It can sometimes give the diagnosis, when history does not help in forming a good hypothesis, e.g., Dix-Hallpike can show BPPV even if history gives no inkling. A complete neurological examination is

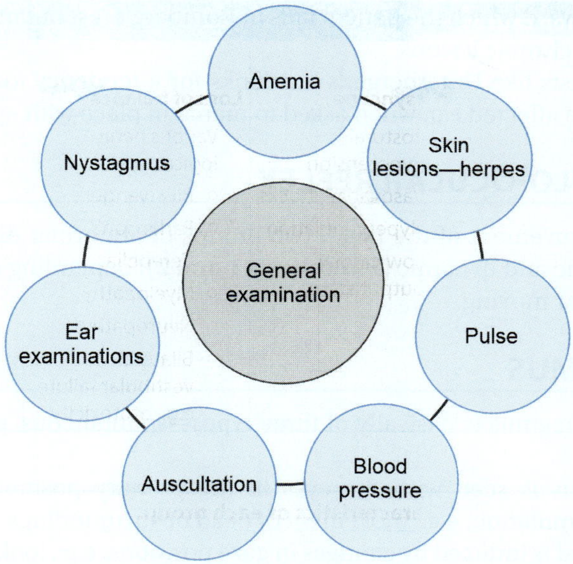

FIG. 1: Schematic representation of general examination in a case of dizziness.

required along with neuro-otological examination in patients with vestibular symptoms.

General Examination

Look for ***(Fig. 1)***:

- Anemia
- *Skin lesions in the ear canal*: To rule out herpes zoster infection.
- *Pulse*: Tachy or bradycardia or an irregular pulse.
- *Blood pressure*: Orthostatic hypotension
- *Auscultation*: Murmurs
- *Ear examinations*: Rinnes and Weber test, eardrum examinations to look for perforation. Hennebert's sign by pushing on the tragus and external auditory meatus to observe if vertigo or nystagmus can be induced.

ASSESSMENTS OF VESTIBULAR FUNCTIONS[3]

Vestibulospinal Reflexes

These are tests that demonstrate the influence of the vestibular system on the spinal cord. Past pointing Romberg's and other tests of posture, and the various walking tests and the gait are the tests in this category.

With an acute vestibular lesion, the patient tilts or might even fall toward the side of the lesion especially with eyes closed. This can be made more sensitive by standing on one's toes or in the tandem position (Sharpened Romberg's test).

Tandem walking with eyes open and eyes closed may show a tendency to fall to one side, but it may occur in cerebellar lesions as well.

The side toward which the patient falls in Romberg's test or tandem walking is not reliable, in chronic lesions.

Stepping tests like Unterberger's test looks for a tendency for the patient to turn toward the affected ear, when asked to march in place with eyes open.

VESTIBULO-OCULAR REFLEX

Based upon movement of the head, two groups of abnormal disturbances are described, static and dynamic **(Flowcharts 1 and 2)**; depending on whether the head is stable or moving.

NYSTAGMUS

Pathologic nystagmus is basically of three types—spontaneous, gaze evoked, or positional.

1. Spontaneous is seen with the eyes in the primary position, without any external stimulation, e.g., movement of head or surroundings.
2. Gaze evoked is induced by changes in gaze positions, e.g., looking to the sides or up or down.
3. Positional nystagmus is not seen at rest or gaze, but seen only in certain positions of the head and body.

To look for pathologic nystagmus, one must examine for nystagmus at rest with and without fixation, in various eye and head positions. Sometimes, pathologic nystagmus may be brought out only after vibration or head shake or hyperventilation. Clinical characteristics are useful to differentiate peripheral from central nystagmus **(Table 6)**.

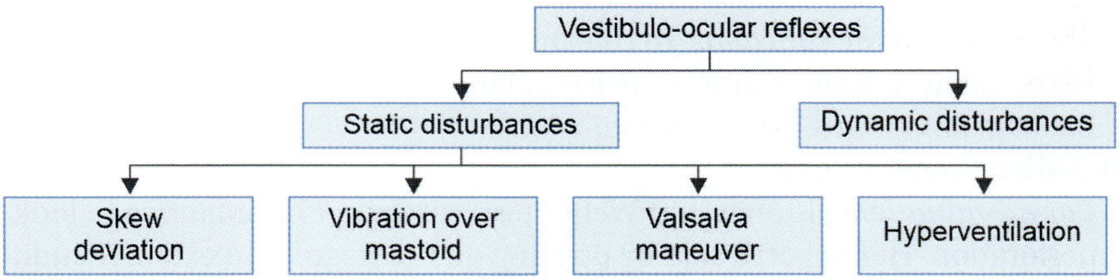

FLOWCHART 1: Vestibulo-ocular reflexes in static head position.

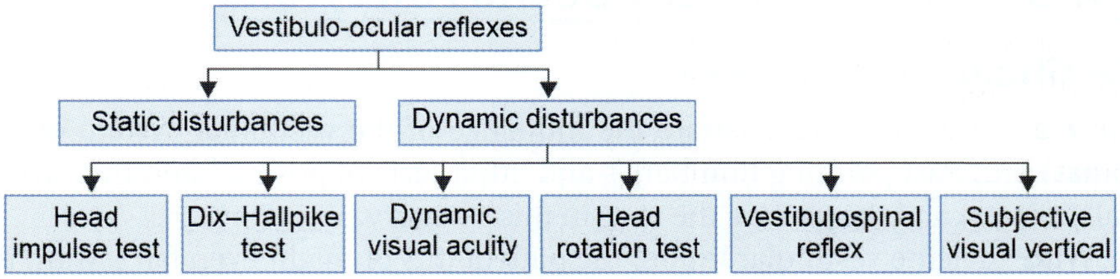

FLOWCHART 2: Vestibulo-ocular reflexes in dynamic head movements.

TABLE 6: Differences between peripheral and central vertigo.

Peripheral nystagmus	Central nystagmus
Unidirectional or mixed	Purely vertical or torsional or direction changing
Reduced by fixation	Not reduced
May follow Alexander's law	Does not follow Alexander's law
Latency present	No latency
Decrease in amplitude	No decrease in amplitude
No fatigability on repeated testing	Fatigability seen
No change in direction of nystagmus	May change in direction
Associated with severe vertigo	Sometimes associated with severe vertigo

Spontaneous Nystagmus

When head is at rest, patient develops nystagmus while looking straight either due to peripheral or central cause.

Alexander's Law

The amplitude of nystagmus increases when the eye moves in the direction of the fast phase (saccades).

Gaze Evoked Nystagmus

Nystagmus changes with gaze position, always due to central pathology. It has three types:

1. Symmetric gaze evoked nystagmus—brainstem or cerebellar disorder.
2. Asymmetric gaze evoked nystagmus—in acoustic neuroma.
3. Dissociated nystagmus—internuclear ophthalmoplegia.

Paroxysmal Positional Nystagmus

Nystagmus seen only in supine or lateral position or Dix-Hallpike maneuver. Both central and peripheral lesions cause paroxysmal positional nystagmus. By this method, able to differentiate BPPV types **(Table 7)**.[4]

Persistent Positional Nystagmus

As long as the provocation position is held, the nystagmus remains. It can be seen in both peripheral lesion like cupulolithiasis variety of BPPV and central lesion like craniovertebral junction anomaly and spinocerebellar degeneration. In central lesion, downbeating variety is seen.

Various Types of Nystagmus

Causes of various types of nystagmus are summarized in **Table 8**.

TABLE 7: Clinical characteristics of benign paroxysmal positional vertigo.

Posterior canal type of BPPV	Horizontal canal type of BPPV[5]	Anterior canal type of BPPV[6]
• Latency of about 3–10 s, rarely lasts >10 s • Upbeating or torsional nystagmus toward affected (downward) ear • Severe vertigo present	• Lasts longer than posterior canal • Horizontal nystagmus on either side (lying supine)-roll test, difficult to diagnose the side • Two types—apogeotropic and geotropic i. Apogeotropic—beating away from earth ii. Geotropic—beating toward earth	• Rare 1–2% maybe more provoked by Dix–Hallpike positioning, to either side • Straight head-hanging position is most sensitive • Diagnostic positioning maneuver cannot identify the side reliably • Nystagmus predominately downbeating with only a small torsional component which points to affected ear • Repositioning needs different maneuvers, like reverse Epley

(BPPV: benign paroxysmal positional vertigo)

TABLE 8: Nystagmus and associated conditions.

Peripheral nystagmus	Labyrinthine disease
Bruns nystagmus	CP angle tumor
Gaze evoked nystagmus:	
Symmetric gaze evoked nystagmus	Brainstem or cerebellar disorders
Asymmetric gaze evoked nystagmus	Acoustic neuroma
Dissociated nystagmus	Multiple sclerosis
Upbeating nystagmus	Multiple sclerosis
Downbeating nystagmus	CV junction anomaly
Pure torsional	Syringomyelia and syringobulbia
Pendular	Congenital and multiple sclerosis
See-saw	Chiasmal lesions
Periodic alternating nystagmus	Congenital and acquired
Persistent positional nystagmus	Apogeotropic benign positional paroxysmal vertigo and central cause

(CP: cerebellopontine; CV: craniovertebral)

SKEW DEVIATION

Skew deviation implies a central pathology and it means vertical misalignment or divergence of the eye.

VIBRATION OF THE MASTOID

Method

Vibrations applied over skull or mastoid brings nystagmus.

Inference

In unilateral lesions, vibration on the mastoid or skull produces nystagmus with slow phase toward paretic ear. If vertical nystagmus is produced, consider central pathology.

HEAD SHAKING NYSTAGMUS

Method

Ask the patient to shake head about 30 times from side to side.

Inference

Nystagmus toward normal side in peripheral pathology, whereas, vertical nystagmus in central pathology.

VALSALVA MANEUVER

Method

Ask the patient to close his mouth, pinching his nose shut, and blow as blowing as balloon, i.e., forceful exhalation against closed glottis.

Inference

Valsalva induced nystagmus almost always peripheral lesions, e.g., superior canal dehiscence, abnormalities in ossicles, oval window, and saccule.

HYPERVENTILATION

Usually, hyperventilation does not produce nystagmus but in case of vestibular nerve demyelination, it is seen, e.g., in multiple sclerosis, vestibular schwannoma.

FRENZEL GOGGLES

The Frenzel goggles are of immense value in the examination of nystagmus, both spontaneously and with various maneuvers. It eliminates fixation and amplifies even minimal nystagmus and one can easily see the effect of various head positions, maneuvers on the nystagmus, e.g., Valsalva maneuver, tragal compression, loud sound, head shake, mastoid vibration, and hyperventilation.

DYNAMIC DISTURBANCES

These disturbances are provoked by head motion or head position change.

HEAD IMPULSE TEST

This is a simple test for identifying vestibular function, described by Halmagyi and Curthoys. Intact vestibular function, with a good VOR, allows the eyes to maintain fixation and keep looking straight at the target despite a sudden unexpected rapid head movement. The VOR makes sure the eyes move rapidly enough to keep the target on the fovea. When the VOR is impaired due to vestibular dysfunction, the eyes get dragged to one side on the sudden head jerk and the patient has to make a corrective saccade to get the eyes back on target.

Method

First grasp the patient face and jaw in both hands and ask the patient to keep looking at a target, e.g., the examiner's nose. Now give a fast head thrust to either side, unpredictably and at various speeds. If the VOR is normal, the patient's eyes remain fixed on the examiner's nose **(Fig. 2)**. But if the VOR is impaired on one side, the eyes get dragged along and the patient has to make a corrective.

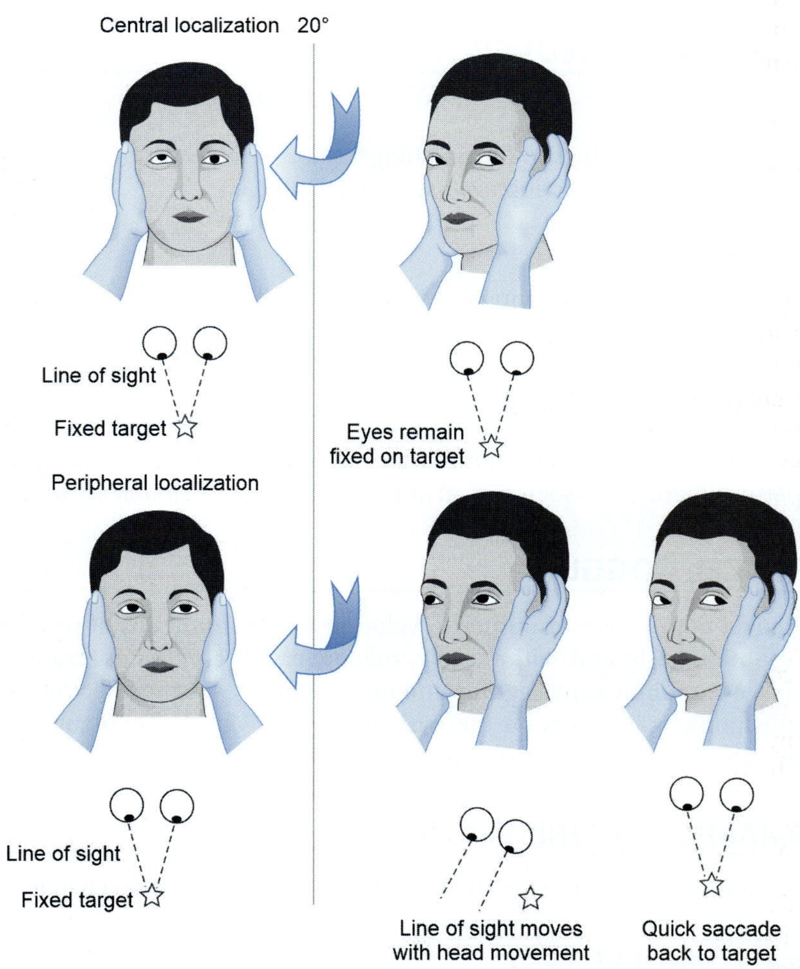

FIG. 2: Head impulse test.

Saccade to get the eyes back to look at the examiner's nose. This refixation saccade can be easily observed at the bedside and is a very important sign of significantly impaired vestibular function on the side to which the head is thrust. The head impulse test (HIT) is almost always positive, in moderate-to-severe paresis of vestibular function. It is almost always positive in acute vestibular neuritis but is usually negative or normal in brainstem or cerebellar infarcts. Thus, in the acute vestibular syndrome, the chances of a brainstem or cerebellar infarct are much more likely, if the HIT is negative. The HIT is usually normal in Ménière's disease, BPPV, or migraine. It may be the only objective sign in bilateral vestibulopathy, e.g., due to aminoglycoside ototoxicity.

DIX–HALLPIKE'S MANEUVER

This test should be done in all patients with history of vertigo, disequilibrium, imbalance, and lightheadedness. It should be done after tests of stance and gait but before caloric and static positional testing. A recent fracture or severe neck or back pain is a relative contraindication.

Method

First, explain the procedure to the patient and obtain consent from the patient. Explain the patient that they may feel dizzy during or after the test and even may vomit. Reassure them that it will be transient. Ask the patients to sit on a couch such that his head will hang down when he lies supine. Inform the patient to keep his eyes in a neutral position and open throughout. Support the patient's head and observe patient's eye during the maneuver. Hold the patient's head, turn it 45° to one side and then make the patient supine, so that head hangs 15–20° below the horizontal. Maintain this position for at least 30–60 seconds and observe nystagmus, if any. Look for latency, direction, duration, fatigability, and habituation, and help the patient sit up and again look for symptoms and nystagmus, then repeat the procedure with head turned 45° to the other side **(Fig. 3)**.

Interpretation

If patient has no nystagmus in sitting, lying on one side with head hanging, then test is completed on that side and repeats the test on other side. If patient has nystagmus then look for latency, direction, duration, and fatigability. The character of the nystagmus in BPPV has been described in the **Table 9**. On bringing the patient back to sitting position, the vertigo recurs with a reversal of nystagmus.

DYNAMIC VISUAL ACUITY

Dynamic visual acuity is a measure of the vestibular function and its performance in maintaining the fixation during active movements of the head. The symptom equivalent of impaired dynamic visual acuity reported in patients with vestibular hypofunction is oscillopsia.

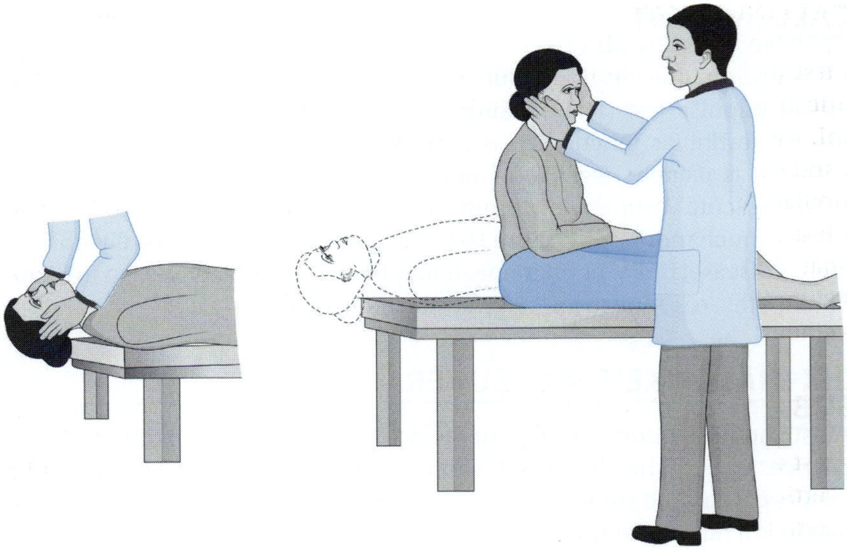

FIG. 3: Dix–Hallpike maneuver.

TABLE 9: Character of the nystagmus in benign paroxysmal positional vertigo (BPPV).

Features of nystagmus	BPPV	Central
Direction	Fixed direction with a mixed rotational, vertical (and a small horizontal component). The fast component of the rotatory component is toward the dependent ear and vertical component is toward the forehead	Changing direction. It may be variable, purely vertical or purely horizontal
Latency	Delay up to 20s before onset	No latency
Fatigability	Fatigability on repeated testing	No fatigability
Habituation	Repeated test produces less response	No habituation

Method

In testing dynamic visual acuity, patient is comfortably seated in a chair. While wearing the corrective glasses, the patient is asked to read the lowest line as possible in the Snellen eye chart. The line with three errors or fewer is considered the lowest line readable. This is recorded as static visual acuity. Now, with the head tilted 30° forward in the pitch plane, the head is turned from side-to-side in the yaw plane at a frequency of 2 Hz. The lowest line readable while the head is in dynamic motion is considered dynamic visual acuity.

Interpretation

A deterioration of acuity of up to two lines in the Snellen eye chart is considered normal. A deterioration of three or more lines in the Snellen eye chart is considered abnormal and is due to hypofunction of the vestibular apparatus. This test has a sensitivity of 55% and a specificity of 100%.

CALORIC TEST

The test is done in both ears, with water at 30–44°C. A rough semiquantitative caloric test, the so called 20-20-20-20 test can also be done. One irrigates 20 mL water at 20°, for 20 seconds, keeping the patients head inclined up at 20°, and notes the duration of nystagmus on either side. The caloric test checks vestibular movements at slow acceleration (<0.5 Hz), while head impulse tests it at fast acceleration (5–10 Hz). So, one might be abnormal when the other is normal. The caloric test in an alert patient can induce uncomfortable vertigo and vomiting. Head impulse is a much more physiological test, since these fast movements are the ones that actually happen in real life.

SUBJECTIVE VISUAL VERTICAL

This test detects abnormal subjective tilt. A normal subject can align a dimly lit bar, vertically with an error of less than one degree to the gravitational vertical. Gravitational vertical is the vertical vector aligned with the gravitational force. This test does not differentiate the central and peripheral lesions. There are several methods to describe this test.

Method

Patient is seated upright with their head fixed in the complete darkness. The patient is asked to set a luminous bar vertically in alignment with the gravitational vertical. The degree of tilt from the gravitational vertical is recorded as the subjective visual vertical (SVV). Optokinetically induced roll vection that is rotated clockwise or counterclockwise in eliciting dynamic SVV results in a greater tilt than the static SVV.

Inference

Ipsiversive deviation of SVV (10–20°) occurs in acute peripheral pathology including utricle and caudal brainstem lesions. Contraversive tilt occurs in upper brainstem lesion. This tilt corresponds to the ocular tilt reaction that occurs in these conditions. The degree of tilt is directly proportional to the severity in peripheral and central vestibular involvement.

How to Diagnose Stroke in Cases of Acute Vestibular Syndrome?

Missing stroke in acute vestibular neuritis leads to catastrophic events in patients and may lead to death. Large posterior fossa hemorrhage needs surgical intervention and close monitoring to prevent death. Proper history taking and neuro-otological and ocular examination differentiate stroke from peripheral etiology; differentiating features are given in **Table 10**.[7]

The combination of these three bedside test collectively called as HINTS.[8] Computed tomography misses 60–90% and magnetic resonance imaging misses up to 30% in acute ischemic posterior circulation strokes.[9]

TABLE 10: Bedside tests to differentiate peripheral and central causes of acute vestibular syndrome.

	Acute vestibular syndromes peripheral	Acute vestibular syndrome central
History	Gradual onset of dizziness	Abrupt onset of dizziness usually vascular etiology
	Positional changes triggers the symptoms	Positional changes may or may not alter the symptoms
Associated symptoms	Nausea with or without vomiting proportionate to the symptoms	May be disproportionate to the symptoms
	No craniocervical pain	Craniocervical pain sometimes present especially in trauma, vertebral artery dissection
	Auditory symptoms usually implies peripheral cause	Acute hearing loss sometimes present in AICA TIA
Risk factors	Viral infections, local pathology	Chronic hypertension, diabetes, cigarette smoking
General neurologic examination	May not differentiate peripheral or central pathology	
Neurovestibular and ocular examination	–	–
Horizontal head impulse test (h-HIT)	Abnormal	Normal but sometimes abnormal in lateral pontine or lateral medullary infarction
Nystagmus	Does not change in direction	May change with direction
Skew deviation	No skew deviation	Skew deviation may be present

(AICA: anterior inferior cerebellar artery; TIA: transient ischemic attack)

HINTS stand for:

- HI: Head impulse test
- N: Nystagmus
- TS: Test for skew deviation.

Reliability of this test is 100%.

This is a rapid bedside examination help to differentiate a stroke mimicking peripheral vestibulopathy, the so called pseudovestibular neuritis presentation of stroke. If this test is positive (any one), central etiology is considered and further evaluation is needed to rule out stroke.

LABORATORY EXAMINATIONS[10]

- Videonystagmography
- Caloric test
- Rotational testing
- Posturography

TiTrATE APPROACH

TiTrATE is the recent consensus approach to a patient with dizziness. It is also called "Triage-TiTrATE-Test", where the TiTrATE stands for timing, triggers, and targeted examination **(Fig. 4)**.[11]

Triage: First, identify whether there are obvious clinical "red flags" that point to a more serious cause for dizziness:

- Abnormal vital signs
- Confusion or otherwise impaired mental state
- Sudden, severe, or sustained head or neck pain
- Worrisome neurologic symptoms (e.g., diplopia, dysarthria, and dysphagia)
- Worrisome cardiovascular symptoms (e.g., chest pain, dyspnea, and syncope)
- Abnormal glucose

If present, these need to be addressed appropriate and urgent manner. It is more useful when encountered with a patient who presents with first time acute onset dizziness.

TiTrATE uses history and examination especially the timing and trigger factors to divide the patients with dizziness into six syndromes. Out of these, four fall into acute presentations and two in chronic presentations. Four acute presentations can be further divide into **(Flowchart 3)**:

- Episodic vestibular syndromes
- Acute vestibular syndromes

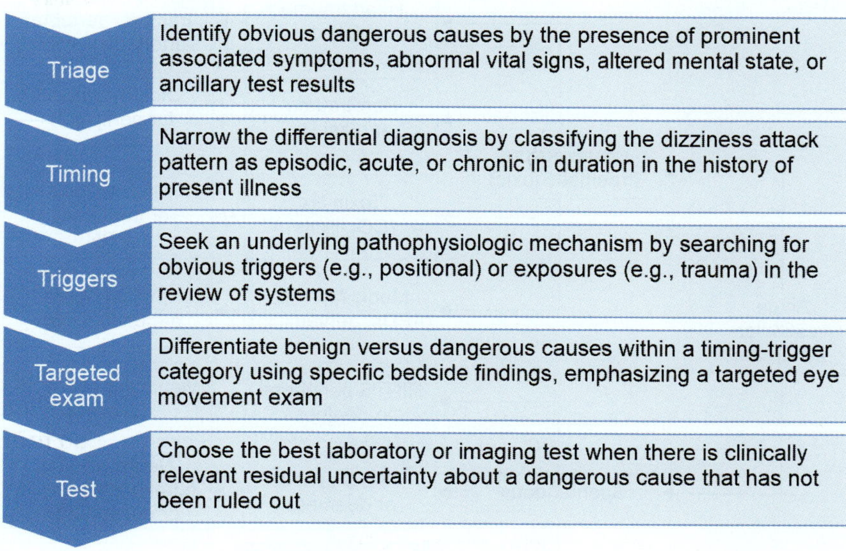

FIG. 4: TiTrATE approach to dizziness.

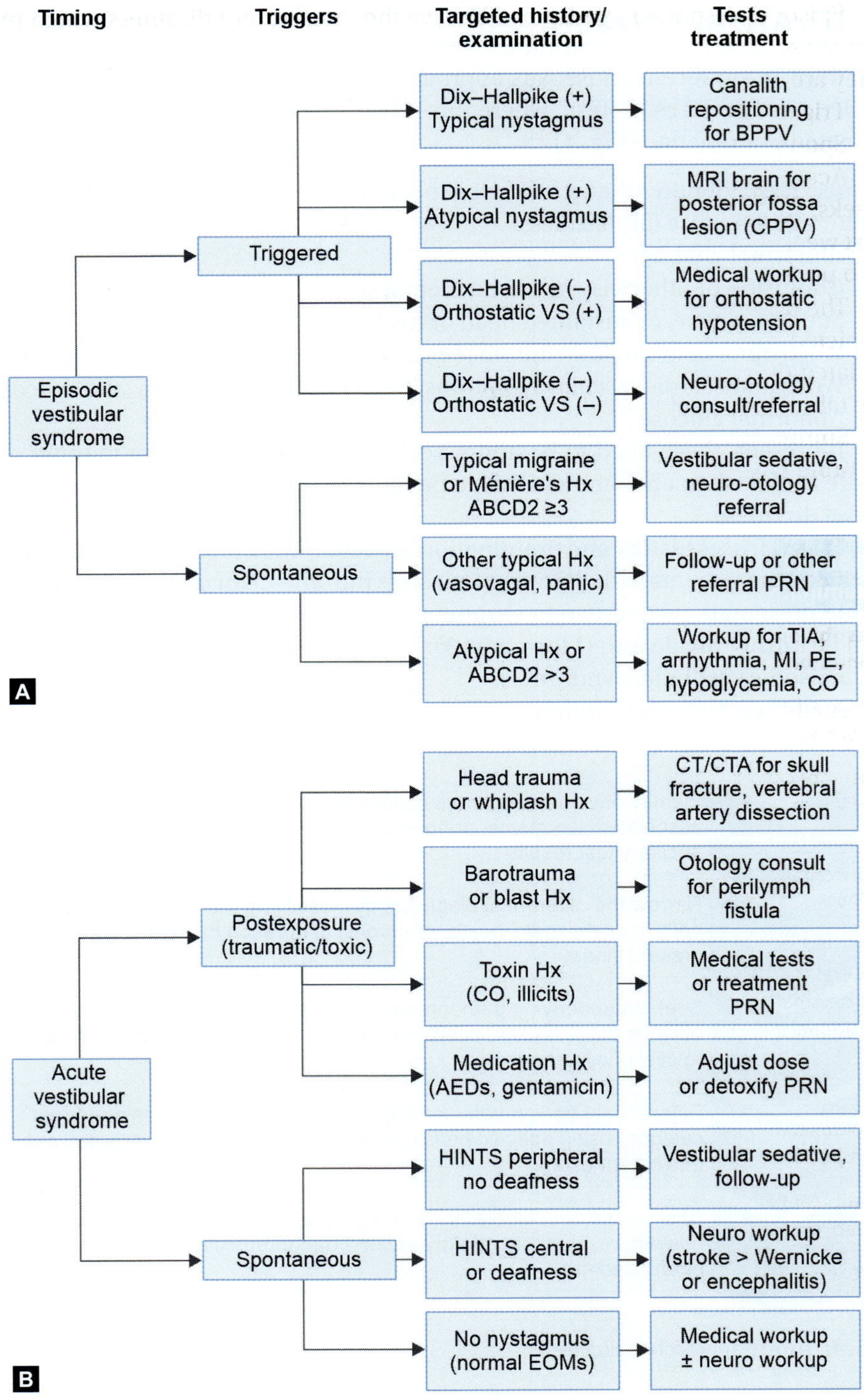

FLOWCHART 3: Classification of vestibular syndrome based on TiTrATE approach.

[AEDs: antiepileptic drugs; CO: carbon monooxide; CPPV: central paroxysmal position al vertigo; CT: computed tomography; CTA: computerized tomographic angiography; EOM: extraocular movement; HINTS: head impulse, nystagmus type, skew; Hx: history; MI: myocardial infarction; PE: pulmonary embolism; PRN: pro re nata (as needed); TIA: transient ischemic attack; VS: vital signs]

Episodic vestibular syndromes involve the intermittent dizziness which may last for seconds, minutes, or hours. Duration of the episode is more important. They are divided into two types:

1. Triggered
2. Spontaneous

Acute vestibular syndromes involve acute, persistent dizziness lasting days to weeks, sometimes with a sequelae. The temporal course at the onset and in the first week is more important than duration. Acute vestibular syndrome is divided into postexposure and spontaneous forms.

The targeted examination and the classification of vestibular syndromes are depicted in **Figure 4** and **Table 11**. Mimickers of benign vestibular causes of isolated dizziness and the safe features to distinguish them from sinister causes are tabulated in **Table 12**.

Summary of the differences between peripheral and central vertigo is shown in **Table 13**.

TABLE 11: Acute vestibular syndromes as per TiTRATE (timing, triggers, and targeted examination) approach.

Vestibular condition	Test maneuver	Nystagmus duration	Trajectory/ Direction	Variation in direction
Triggered episodic vestibular syndrome (episodic nystagmus triggered by specific positional maneuvers)				
Posterior canal BPPV	Head hanging with 45° turn to each side (Dix–Hallpike)	5–30 s	Upbeat-torsional	Direction reversal on arising
Horizontal canal BPPV	Supine roll to either side (Pagnini–McClure)	30–90 s	Horizontal	Spontaneous reversal during test
Central paroxysmal positional vertigo	Any (usually head hanging)	5–60 s (sometimes persistent if position is held)	Any (usually downbeat or horizontal)	Any (often direction-fixed)
Spontaneous acute vestibular syndrome (spontaneous nystagmus that may be exacerbated nonspecifically by various head maneuvers)				
Vestibular neuritis or labyrinthitis	Gaze testing	Persistent	Dominantly horizontal	Direction-fixed (acutely)
Stroke	Gaze testing	Persistent	Any (usually dominantly horizontal, occasionally vertical or torsional)	Direction-fixed or direction-changing with gaze position

TABLE 12: Mimickers and safe to go features for the benign vestibular causes of isolated dizziness.

Syndrome	Targeted examination	Benign disorder	Dangerous mimic	"Safe-to-go" features
t-EVS	Orthostatic vitals; positional tests for nystagmus	BPPV	Posterior fossa mass	• No pain, auditory, neurologic symptoms, or syncope • Symptoms not limited to arising and occur when tipping head forward/back or rolling in bed • Asymptomatic with head stationary, symptoms reproduced by specific positional tests **(Table 3)** • Characteristic, canal-specific, peripheral-type nystagmus on positional tests **(Table 3)** • Therapeutic response to canal-specific repositioning maneuvers [posterior canal: Modified Epley maneuver; horizontal canal: Lempert roll (barbecue) maneuver]
s-EVS	Head, neck, and cranial nerve history; ear, hearing history	Vestibular migraine or Ménière's disease	TIA	• No cardiorespiratory symptoms or transient loss of consciousness • No diplopia or other "Dangerous D" symptoms (dysarthria, dysphagia, dysphonia, and dysmetria) • No papilledema, Horner's syndrome, cranial nerve signs (e.g., facial palsy) [especially if headache present] • No sudden, severe, or sustained pain (especially located in the posterior neck) • Strong/long past history of dizziness episodes (at least 5 spells over >2 years) • Clear precipitants (e.g., stress, food, and visual motion) for multiple episodes or ABCD2 risk score ≤3 • *Migraine*: History of migraine headache; classic visual aura or photophobia with most attacks • *Menière's*: History of unilateral fluctuating hearing loss or tinnitus with most attacks

Continued

Continued

Syndrome	Targeted examination	Benign disorder	Dangerous mimic	"Safe-to-go" features
s-AVS	HINTS; ear, hearing exam	Vestibular neuritis	Stroke	• Maximum 1 prodromal spell <48 h before onset • No excessive vomiting or gait disorder • No pain, auditory, neurologic symptoms • No papilledema, Horner's syndrome, cranial nerve signs (e.g., facial palsy) [especially if headache present] • Stands and walks unassisted (even if unsteady or wide-based) • HINTS plus hearing/ear examination–"SENDHIMONHOME"96 ○ SEND—Straight eyes (no vertical ocular misalignment a.k.a. "skew"), no Deafness ○ HIM—Head Impulse Misses (unilateral abnormal impulse opposite nystagmus direction) ○ ON—One-way Nystagmus (unidirectional nystagmus worse in gaze toward fastphase) ○ HOME—Healthy Otic and Mastoid Exam (pearly tympanic membrane with no pimples, pus, or perforation; no pain on palpation of the mastoid)

(t-EVS: triggered episodic vestibular syndrome; s-AVS: spontaneous acute vestibular syndrome; s-EVS: spontaneous episodic vestibular syndromes; TIA: transient ischemic attack; HINTS: head impulse, nystagmus type, skew; BPPV: benign paroxysmal positional vertigo)

TABLE 13: Summary of the differences between peripheral and central vertigo.

Peripheral vertigo	Central vertigo
Spontaneous nystagmus—unidirectional, mixed	Pure vertical or torsional or changing direction
No gaze evoked nystagmus	Gaze evoked nystagmus present
Latency and fatigability seen in paroxysmal, positional nystagmus	No latent period, no fatigability
No skew deviation	Skew deviation implies central lesion
Vibration over the mastoid—slow phase toward paretic ear	Vertical nystagmus
Valsalva maneuver indicates peripheral lesion	Not present
Hyperventilation-slow phase towards paretic ear	Excitatory nystagmus
Head impulse test—abnormal	Normal
Dix–Hallpike's—positive	Negative
Dynamic visual acuity—labyrinthine dysfunction	–
Subjective visual vertical does not differentiate central and peripheral lesion	–

CONCLUSION

Dizziness and vertigo are very common syndromes in daily practice. A systematic history followed by a hypothesis generation is the first and foremost step for approaching any case of dizziness. Examination is the vital step which can confirm the diagnosis and in situations where the history is not clear will only be the physician's tool for diagnosis. In an acute vestibular syndrome, the TiTrATE approach is helpful to rule out more serious cause and HINTS is helpful to diagnose a stroke in such cases. Proceeding to investigate a case without the history and examination might end-up missing the common causes or unwantedly investigating an incidental finding. Therefore, clinical examination still stands as the gold standard in approaching a case of giddiness.

REFERENCES

1. Kerber KA, Meurer WJ, West BT, Fendrick AM. Dizziness presentations in U.S. emergency departments, 1995-2004. Acad Emerg Med. 2008;15(8):744-50.
2. Karatas M. Central vertigo and dizziness: epidemiology, differential diagnosis, and common causes. Neurologist. 2008;14(6):355-64.
3. Baloh RW, Kerber KA. Clinical neurophysiology of the vestibular system. In: Contemporary Neurology Series, 4th edition. New York: Oxford University Press; 2011.
4. Nakayama M, Epley JM. BPPV and variants: improved treatment results with automated, nystagmus-based repositioning. Otolaryngol Head Neck Surg. 2005;133(1):107-12.
5. Cakir BO, Ercan I, Cakir ZA, Civelek S, Sayin I, Turgut S. What is the true incidence of horizontal semicircular canal benign paroxysmal positional vertigo? Otolaryngol Head Neck Surg. 2006;134(3):451-4.
6. Jackson LE, Morgan B, Fletcher JC Jr, Krueger WW. Anterior canal benign paroxysmal positional vertigo: an underappreciated entity. Otol Neurotol. 2007;28(2):218-22.
7. Newman-Toker DE. Acute vestibular syndrome. [online] Available from www.content.lib.utah.edu/utils/getfile/collection/ehsl-dent/id/7/filename/5.pdf [Last accessed March, 2025].
8. Kattah JC, Talkad AV, Wang DZ, Hsieh YH, Newman-Toker DE. HINTS to diagnose stroke in the acute vestibular syndrome: three-step bedside oculomotor examination more sensitive than early MRI diffusion-weighted imaging. Stroke. 2009;40(11):3504-10.
9. Edlow JA, Newman-Toker DE, Savitz SI. Diagnosis and initial management of cerebellar infarction. Lancet Neurol. 2008;7(10):951-64
10. British Audiology Society. [online] Available from http://www.thebsa.org.uk/ [Last accessed March, 2025].
11. David E. Newman-Toker, Jonathan A. Edlow TiTrATE: A novel approach to diagnosing acute dizziness and vertigo. Neurol Clin. 2015;33(3):577-99.

4 CHAPTER Eye Movements in Vertigo

Shaik Farheen Bhanu, Kranthi Karunakaran, Sundar Shanmugam

ABSTRACT

Vertigo is a common presenting complaint in primary care and emergency departments. The affected individuals most often present with eye movement abnormalities. Its etiology could range from a simple peripheral vestibular cause like BPPV, Ménière's to more severe central causes like posterior circulation strokes and brainstem syndromes. The vestibular system helps to maintain balance during head movement, dysfunction of this causes the brain to misinterpret the asymmetry resulting in vertigo and a compensatory vestibular nystagmus. Brainstem contains the centers for horizontal gaze in the pons and vertical gaze in the midbrain and the accuracy of eye movements is ultimately coordinated by the cerebellum. Damage to these centers respectively causes horizontal or vertical nystagmus and loss of saccadic accuracy. Hence, a careful examination of eye movements plays a crucial role in localizing various vertigo related disorders to central or peripheral causes. This chapter provides a systematic approach to the various eye movements and their abnormalities that can help to diagnose the cause and provide optimal targeted treatment.

INTRODUCTION

Abnormalities in eye movements are a frequent and prominent finding in diseases causing Vertigo. However, it gains little attention as patients themselves do not always complain about visual symptoms. Hence, careful oculomotor examination is paramount in the evaluation of a patient with vertigo. Recognizing and capturing these abnormal eye movements helps in the diagnosis and differential diagnosis of vertigo-related disorders. This chapter presents a comprehensive review about various eye movement abnormalities that are commonly found in vertigo.

NORMAL EYE MOVEMENTS

Eye movements are primarily classified into two categories—those that maintain image stability on the fovea—such as fixation, smooth pursuit, the vestibulo-ocular reflex, and optokinetic reflexes—and those that redirect the fovea's focus to a different area.[1]

Saccades

Saccades are quick, coordinated eye movements that shift the line of sight between different points of fixation. To evaluate them, the patient is asked to look alternately between two targets, such as the examiner's nose and the tip of a pen. These movements are assessed in both horizontal and vertical planes, with attention given to their speed, precision, and synchronization.[2,3]

Smooth Pursuit

Smooth pursuit refers to slow, continuous eye movements that enable the fovea to maintain focus on a moving object. During testing, the patient is instructed to track a target moving at a steady pace in horizontal and vertical directions while keeping the head still. If the eyes fail to match the target's motion precisely, corrective catch-up saccades may occur.[4,5]

Vestibulo-ocular Reflex

During routine activities, head movements involve both angular rotation and linear acceleration. The oculomotor system ensures gaze stabilization in space by utilizing the vestibulo-ocular reflex (VOR) and the ocular counter-rolling reflex. The VOR functions by generating compensatory eye movements in the opposite direction of head motion, thereby stabilizing the visual field and preserving a steady retinal image.[6]

Optokinetic Nystagmus

Optokinetic nystagmus is triggered by continuous environmental motion, such as the view passing by when looking out of a moving car. It allows the eyes to maintain focus on a moving object or scene as it traverses the visual field. This response consists of alternating smooth pursuit movements and corrective saccades, complementing the VOR to sustain stable vision during prolonged movement.

Vergence

Vergence movements adjust eye alignment to maintain focus on objects that shift in depth relative to the observer. This mechanism ensures that both eyes remain directed at a target as its distance changes.

ABNORMAL EYE MOVEMENTS

For clear and stable vision, a visual target must be accurately positioned and maintained on the fovea, the area of the retina with the highest density of cone photoreceptors and the greatest visual acuity. This stability is ensured by three primary mechanisms:

- *Fixation stabilization*, which relies on visual feedback processes to suppress unwanted saccades and correct retinal drifts through programmed eye movements.

- *VORs,* which help maintain eye position despite minor head and body movements.
- *Neural integrators,* which counteract the natural elastic pull of orbital tissues, allowing the eyes to sustain eccentric gaze positions without drifting back to the center.[7]

These mechanisms form the physiological basis for understanding nystagmus and saccadic intrusions, along with the symptoms they may cause.

Nystagmus and saccadic intrusions are both involuntary eye movements that may be either pathological or part of normal physiology. These movements often present as repetitive oscillations, disrupting steady fixation. When occurring in the primary gaze, they displace the fovea from the intended target, resulting in retinal image instability, which can lead to oscillopsia (the sensation of a moving visual field) and diminished visual acuity. Nystagmus is characterized by rhythmic, continuous movements that persist in the central gaze, whereas saccadic intrusions are irregular, episodic, and transient. The key distinction between the two lies in the initiating movement: Nystagmus begins with a slow drifting phase, while saccadic intrusions are initiated by abrupt, rapid eye movements.[8]

Nystagmus

Nystagmus refers to involuntary, rhythmic eye movements that can be congenital or acquired. It is broadly classified into jerk nystagmus and pendular nystagmus, both of which can have horizontal, vertical, or torsional components. In jerk nystagmus, the eyes drift slowly away from the intended position, followed by a rapid corrective movement. While the slow phase reflects the underlying pathology, the fast phase determines the nystagmus' direction. In pendular nystagmus, the slow drift is followed by continuous to-and-fro slow oscillations.

Saccadic Intrusions

Saccadic intrusions refer to unwanted saccadic eye movements that disrupt steady fixation. These involuntary movements are initiated by fast saccades that momentarily displace the eyes from central fixation and are often triggered by gaze shifts. Unlike saccadic dysmetria, where the eyes overshoot or undershoot an intended target, saccadic intrusions arise spontaneously. They are categorized based on the presence or absence of an intersaccadic interval. Those with an interval include square-wave jerks, macrosquare wave jerks, and macrosaccadic oscillations, whereas ocular flutter and opsoclonus occur without an intersaccadic interval.

Saccadic Abnormalities

Peripheral vestibular disorders do not influence saccadic eye movements. Horizontal saccades slow down when the paramedian pontine reticular formation (PPRF) is affected, whereas vertical saccadic slowing occurs due to damage to the rostral interstitial nucleus of the medial longitudinal fasciculus (MLF). In general, pontine lesions predominantly affect horizontal saccades, while midbrain lesions impair vertical ones. Additionally, saccades may be inaccurate, either overshooting (hypermetria) or undershooting (hypometria) their target, requiring corrective adjustments. Such dysmetric saccades often result from cerebellar dysfunction, particularly involving the dorsal vermis or its related neural circuits.[9,10]

Pursuit Abnormalities

Smooth pursuit eye movements rely on multiple neural structures, making it difficult to pinpoint a lesion solely based on impaired pursuit. However, a significant asymmetry in smooth pursuit suggests a unilateral lesion affecting the pursuit pathway. In patients with horizontal nystagmus, the pursuit may be impaired in the direction of the nystagmus, making vertical pursuit testing useful in evaluating acute vestibular dysfunction.

Vestibulo-ocular Reflex Abnormalities

A functioning VOR generates compensatory eye movements opposite to head rotation, keeping the gaze stable. In patients with peripheral vestibular dysfunction, a head impulse toward the affected side results in a catch-up saccade at the end of head movement, indicating reduced VOR gain. In contrast, a normal head impulse test in a patient with acute vertigo and spontaneous nystagmus suggests a central vestibular pathology. Additionally, if a refixation saccade occurs in an unexpected plane (e.g., a vertical saccade following a horizontal rotation), it may indicate a central lesion.[11,12]

Optokinetic Nystagmus Abnormalities

Asymmetries in optokinetic nystagmus (OKN) can help localize visual field deficits. While postchiasmal lesions can cause homonymous hemianopia, occipital lobe lesions typically preserve OKN, whereas parietal lesions affecting the optic radiations disrupt OKN responses when stimuli move toward the side of the lesion.

Vergence Abnormalities

Vergence dysfunction leads to horizontal ocular misalignment at specific distances, causing binocular diplopia during near or distant viewing. Patients may perceive a slight oblique misorientation, though the primary deviation remains horizontal. Both convergence and divergence dysfunction may occur as either paresis or spasm, resulting in varying misalignment at different viewing distances.

PERIPHERAL VESTIBULAR DISORDERS

The vestibular system maintains a continuous baseline firing rate, known as vestibular tone. When the head moves, signals from one vestibular labyrinth increase above this resting rate, while those from the opposite side decrease, creating a push-pull dynamic that enhances motion detection. Disruptions to this balance, such as damage to one labyrinth, can lower its firing rate, leading the brain to misinterpret the asymmetry as an unintended motion.[13] This results in vertigo and compensatory vestibular nystagmus, typically exhibiting both horizontal and torsional components. Because central gaze-stabilizing mechanisms remain functional, visual fixation can often suppress or reduce the nystagmus.

CENTRAL VESTIBULAR DISORDERS

Central vestibular dysfunctions are categorized based on their anatomic location within the brainstem or cerebellum.[14]

Brainstem Contributions to Gaze Control—the Pons

The pons and rostral medulla regulate horizontal gaze, with the abducens nucleus serving as the center for conjugating horizontal eye movements. This nucleus contains:

- Motor neurons that control the lateral rectus muscle.
- Internuclear neurons that project across the midline via the MLF to activate the contralateral medial rectus muscle.

Lesions affecting the abducens nucleus may impair horizontal gaze toward the affected side. However, vergence movements (which allow for focusing on near objects) remain intact since they bypass this pathway.

Damage to the MLF results in internuclear ophthalmoplegia (INO), characterized by slowed or restricted adduction of the affected eye. The VOR for horizontal head movements relies on signals from the lateral semicircular canals, which transmit input to the contralateral abducens nucleus via the medial vestibular nucleus (MVN). Conditions such as Wernicke's encephalopathy, which affects chronic alcoholics due to thiamine deficiency, can disrupt the vestibular nuclei and impair horizontal VOR. Additionally, the PPRF sends signals to the abducens nucleus for horizontal saccades. Lesions in this region result in slow or absent horizontal saccadic movements.

The nucleus prepositus hypoglossi (NPH) and the adjacent MVN, influenced by the cerebellum, are responsible for maintaining an eccentric gaze (holding the eyes to the far right or left). This system functions by integrating visual, vestibular, and saccadic signals. Impairment of this network—due to cerebellar pathology or alcohol intoxication—causes the eyes to drift back to the center, resulting in gaze-evoked nystagmus.

Brainstem Contributions to Gaze Control—the Midbrain

The midbrain is critical for vertical gaze control and vergence eye movements. The oculomotor and trochlear nuclei contain motor neurons responsible for:

- Vertical eye movements (via the superior and inferior rectus muscles).
- Torsional eye rotations (via the superior and inferior oblique muscles).

The rostral interstitial nucleus of the riMLF provides the necessary input for vertical saccades. Bilateral riMLF lesions, as seen in progressive supranuclear palsy (PSP), lead to slow or absent vertical saccades.

Unilateral riMLF lesions, caused by rostral brainstem strokes or hypothalamic hamartomas, result in loss of torsional quick phases, causing the top pole of the eye to rotate toward the side of the lesion.

Signals for vertical vestibular and pursuit eye movements travel from the medulla and pons to the midbrain via the MLF. Bilateral MLF lesions, such as those in multiple sclerosis, impair vertical smooth pursuit and vestibular responses, along with bilateral adduction failure during horizontal saccades. The interstitial nucleus of Cajal (INC) is crucial for maintaining a vertical eccentric gaze (such as looking upward for extended periods). Damage to this nucleus results in gaze-evoked nystagmus in the upward or downward direction due to a faulty ocular motor integrator. The INC is also involved in head movement control, and dysfunction can cause abnormal head posturing and twisting movements.

CEREBELLAR CONTRIBUTIONS TO GAZE CONTROL

Three regions of the cerebellum play distinct roles in eye movement regulation:[15-17]

1. *Flocculus and paraflocculus*: These structures are essential for smooth pursuit, eccentric gaze holding, and VOR adaptation to maintain clear vision during head motion.
   Lesions result in downbeat nystagmus, commonly observed in Chiari malformation and hereditary spinocerebellar ataxias (e.g., episodic ataxia type 2).
2. *Nodulus and ventral uvula*: These regions regulate velocity storage, sustaining vestibular nystagmus even after head movement has ceased. Lesions here produce periodic alternating nystagmus, where horizontal nystagmus reverses direction approximately every 2 minutes.
   The nodulus also contributes to the brain's gravitational force estimation, influencing vestibular ocular reflex axis modulation. Dysfunction can lead to central positional nystagmus.
3. *Dorsal vermis and fastigial nucleus*:
   These structures ensure saccadic accuracy:
   - Dorsal vermis lesions cause saccadic hypometria (undershooting of targets).
   - Fastigial nucleus lesions result in saccadic hypermetria (overshooting). The fastigial nucleus sends crossed projections, meaning lesions cause bilateral saccadic hypermetria.[18]
   - Wallenberg's syndrome (lateral medullary infarction) disrupts this balance, causing lateropulsion of saccadic movements (overshooting toward the lesion side, undershooting away from it).

CONCLUSION

This article summarizes the current models of normal eye movements. Knowing these abnormal eye movements may help in the identification of specific diseases causing vertigo. A systemic approach to examination of the abnormal eye movements has been emphasized so that diagnosis is optimal and correct.

REFERENCES

1. John RJ, Zee DS. The Neurology of Eye Movements, 4th edition. New York: Oxford University Press; 2006.
2. Leigh RJ, Kennard C. Using saccades as a research tool in the clinical neurosciences. Brain. 2004;127(Pt 3):460-7.
3. Ramat S, Leigh RJ, Zee DS, Optican LM. Ocular oscillations are generated by the coupling of brainstem excitatory and inhibitory saccadic burst neurons. Exp Brain Res. 2005;160(1): 89-106.
4. Sung KB, Lee TK, Furman JM. Abnormal Eye Movements in Dizzy Patients. Neurol Clin. 2005;23(3):675-703.
5. Kang JJ, Choi S, Na S, Oh SY. Recording and interpretation of ocular movements: spontaneous and induced nystagmus. 2023;25(1):10-8.
6. Kheradmand A, Colpak AI, Zee DS. Eye movements in vestibular disorders. Handb Clin Neurol. 2016;137:103-17.
7. Beh SC, Frohman TC, Frohman EM. Cerebellar Control of Eye Movements. J Neuro-ophthalmol. 2017;37(1):87-98.
8. Strupp M, Kremmyda O, Adamczyk C, Böttcher N, Muth C, Yip CW, et al. Central ocular motor disorders, including gaze palsy and nystagmus. J Neurol. 2014;261Suppl 2(Suppl 2):S542-58.
9. Büttner U, Straube A. The effect of cerebellar midline lesions on eye movements. Neuro-ophthalmol. 1995;15:75-82.
10. Zee DS, Yamazaki A, Butler PH, Gücer G. Effects of ablation of flocculus and paraflocculus of eye movements in primate. J Neurophysiol. 1981;46(4):878-99.
11. Baloh RW, Honrubia V, Yee RD, Hess K. Changes in the human vestibulo-ocular reflex after loss of peripheral sensitivity. Ann Neurol. 1984;16(2):222-8.
12. Baloh RH, Honrubia V. The vestibular system; in Baloh RH, Honrubia V (Eds): Clinical Neurophysiology of the Vestibular System, 2nd edition. Philadelphia: FA Davis; 1990. pp. 1-17.
13. Galiana HL, Guitton D. Central organization and modeling of eye-head coordination during orienting gaze shifts. Ann N Y Acad Sci. 1992;656:452-71.
14. Krauzlis RJ. The control of voluntary eye movements: new perspectives. Neuroscientist. 2005;11(2):124-37.
15. Blazquez PM, Hirata Y, Highstein SM. The vestibulo-ocular reflex as a model system for motor learning: what is the role of the cerebellum? Cerebellum. 2004;3(3):188-92.
16. Enderle JD, Engelken EJ. Effects of cerebellar lesions on saccade simulations. Biomed Sci Instrum. 1996;32:13-21.
17. Porrill J, Warren PA, Dean P. A simple control law generates Listing's positions in a detailed model of the extraocular muscle system. Vision Res. 2000;40(27):3743-58.
18. Glasauer S. Cerebellar contribution to saccades and gaze holding: a modeling approach. Ann NY Acad Sci. 2003;1004:206-19.

5 CHAPTER

Investigating Vertigo: Laboratory Testing and Neuroimaging

Balasubramanian Samivel, Lenin S Palanisamy, Saranya Masilamani, Lakshmi Narasimhan Ranganathan, Gobinathan Shankar

ABSTRACT

Vertigo is one of the most common and disabling complaints that a physician comes across in his daily practice. But, most of these patients do not undergo a detailed laboratory investigation except for neuroimaging. The possible reasons for this underutilization could be lack of exposure, consumption of time, and nonavailability. But, these tests do have a definite role in the management of a dizzy patient which cannot be done with clinical examination alone. This chapter discusses the role of both the tests for functional integrity and tests for structural integrity of the vestibular system. These tests will help us to localize the site of lesion and to know about the nature of lesion and thus aids in the management of dizzy patients.

INTRODUCTION

Vertigo as defined by the currently used International classification of vestibular disorders is "the sensation of self-motion when no self-motion is occurring or the sensation of distorted self-motion during an otherwise normal head movement."[1] It will be more distressing to the patient as the perception of self in space is distorted. It is crucial to differentiate between vertigo and other causes of dizziness because the pathophysiology differs, and hence, the management. It is equally important to differentiate between central and peripheral vertigo and the possible etiologies of each because the management of each differs and some of them may be alarming and deserve immediate medical attention and some may be innocuous and may need only reassurance. Despite these, patients with vertigo rarely ever undergo laboratory evaluation because of the lack of availability of the facilities and due to lack of exposure of the treating physician to these tests. Even though these laboratory tests cannot replace a good clinical history and a dedicated clinical examination, they do compliment the conventional clinical examination in various ways. For example, the sensitivity of electronystagmography (ENG) or video-oculography (VOG) is high when compared to the clinical tests alone, and the sensitivity increases further when combined with clinical maneuver. Some of these tests may have prognostic value as auditory brainstem response (ABR) has in brainstem stroke.[2] The laboratory investigations most commonly used in evaluation of vertigo are discussed in this chapter.

The various investigations available for the evaluation of vestibular disorders can be grossly classified into:
- Functional tests
- Structural tests

Functional tests can be further classified into:
- Tests for semicircular canals
- Tests for otolith organs
- Test for multilevel localization
- Tests for functional integrity of the vestibular system which includes vestibular evoked myogenic potentials (VEMP), ENG, VOG, neuro-orthoptic procedure-subjective visual vertical (SVV) testing, gait analysis, posturography, pure tone audiometry, and auditory ABR.
- Tests for structural integrity of the vestibular system namely neuroimaging.

TESTS FOR FUNCTIONAL INTEGRITY OF VESTIBULAR SYSTEM

Vestibular Evoked Myogenic Potentials

The very first person to observe the responsiveness of the vestibular system to auditory stimulus was Von Bekesy whose work formed the basis of VEMP. Even though many pioneers in the field of neuro-otology recorded short latent responses from various parts of scalp, it was Colebatch et al. who first recorded short latency myogenic potentials from sternocleidomastoid following stimulation with brief clicks.

Later, similar myogenic potentials were also recorded from the extraocular muscles, masseter, trapezius, and splenius capitis. Among these, cervical-VEMP (cVEMP) and ocular-VEMP (oVEMP) are in clinical use.

Origin of Vestibular Evoked Myogenic Potentials

Vestibular stimulation with various stimuli (usually tone bursts but also skull tap, vibration, and galvanic current) results in the activation of vestibulocollicular pathway (for cVEMP) and vestibulo-ocular pathway (for oVEMP) producing an inhibitory potential in sternocleidomastoid and extraocular muscles, respectively, which are recorded by the surface electrodes **(Flowcharts 1 and 2)**.

The cVEMP done with air conducted tone burst stimulus is essentially a test for saccule and inferior vestibular nerve whereas the utricle and superior vestibular nerve are essential in the generation of oVEMPS.[3]

CLINICAL RELEVANCE OF VESTIBULAR EVOKED MYOGENIC POTENTIALS

This test identifies the intactness of the cVEMP and oVEMP **(Fig. 1)**.

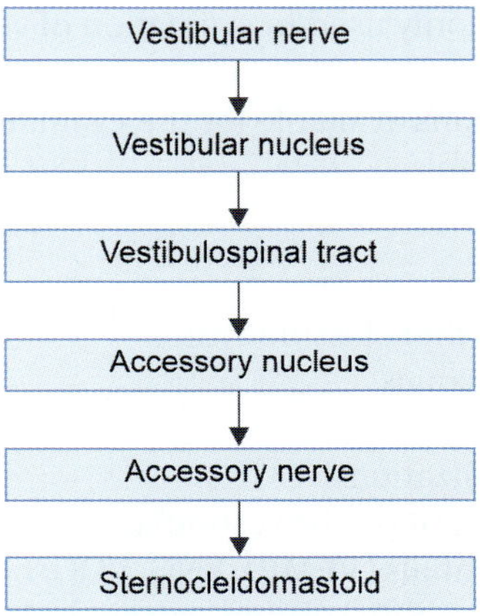

FLOWCHART 1: Vestibulo-collicular pathway.

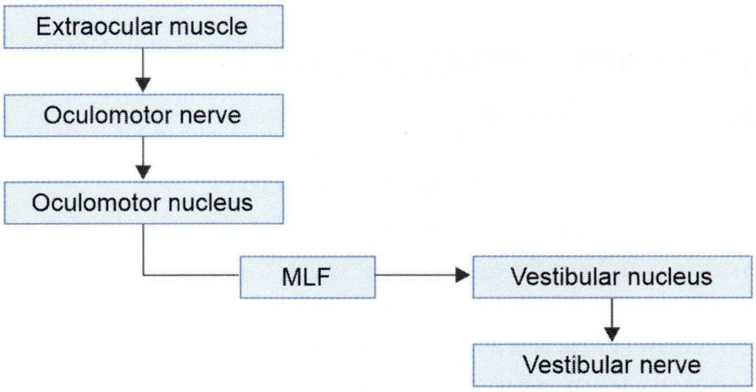

FLOWCHART 2: Vestibulo-ocular pathway.

(MLF: medial longitudinal fasciculus).

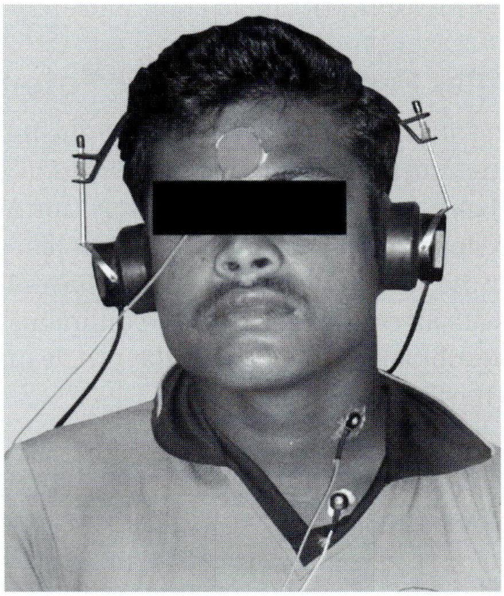

FIG. 1: Testing set-up for vestibular evoked myogenic potentials.

Test Procedure

Prerequisites

Normal conductive apparatus of the ear with air-bone gap of <20 dB.

The test can be done both in supine and sitting posture but preferably be done in sitting position in view of technical feasibility. The active electrode is placed over the middle of the sternocleidomastoid muscle belly. The indifferent electrode is placed over the tendinous insertion of the muscle at the clavicle. The most important part of the test is the tonic contraction of the sternocleidomastoid muscle. The force exerted on both sides should be approximately equal because the amplitude is directly proportional to the level of contraction. This can be easily done by asking the patient to give resistance against an inflated blood pressure cuff while simultaneously monitoring the deflection of needle in the manometer.

The responses to be noted are latency of the waves, amplitudes of the positive and negative peaks at 13th millisecond and 23rd millisecond, respectively (P13 and N23) **(Fig. 2)**.

Crossed excitation is inhibitory myogenic response from the contralateral sternocleidomastoid muscle with opposite polarity but with same latency.

Results and their Interpretation

In general, absence of both the components or decreased amplitudes of the components indicates a peripheral pathology whereas prolonged latencies indicate central pathology.

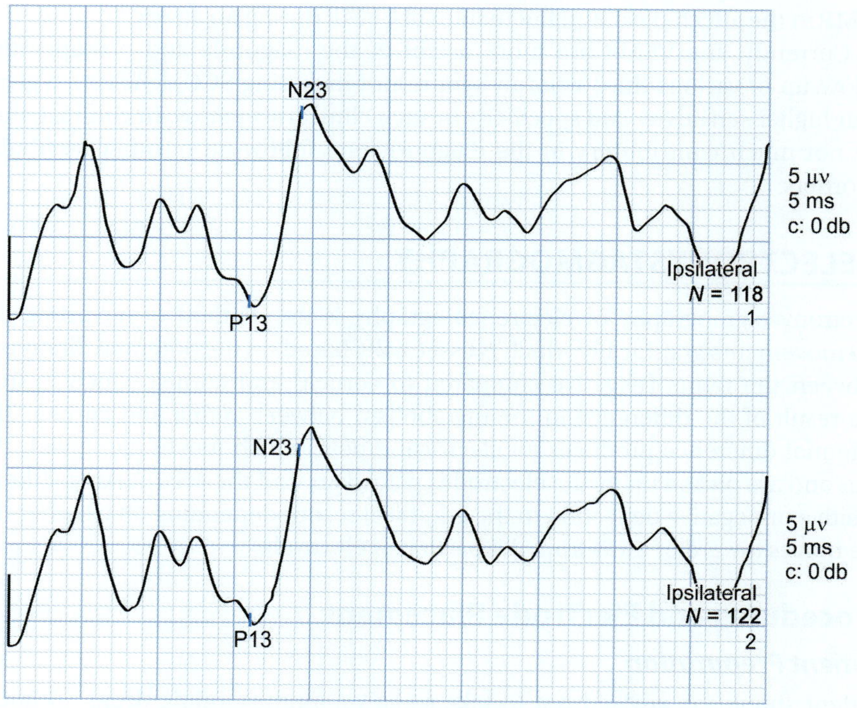

FIG. 2: Normal waveforms of vestibular evoked myogenic potentials.

Amplitude asymmetry ratio: Compared to absolute values of amplitude, amplitude asymmetry ratio increases the reliability.

$$\text{Amplitude asymmetry ratio} = L - R/L + R \times 100$$

It is considered abnormal when the value is >35%.

Large amplitude, low threshold response indicates the presence of a 3rd window [superior semicircular canal (SCC) dehiscence].

A discrepancy between the oVEMP and cVEMP helps us to localize the lesion within brainstem. For example, presence of normal cVEMP with an abnormal oVEMP indicate a pathology in pons and midbrain whereas an abnormal cVEMP with normal oVEMP indicate lesion in medulla.

VESTIBULAR EVOKED MYOGENIC POTENTIALS IN SPECIFIC VESTIBULAR DISORDERS

Vestibulocollicular pathway amplitudes are abnormal in patients with vestibular schwannoma, which may be absent or delayed. It is seen in 80% of patients according to Murofushi et al.

In case of acute vestibular neuritis, the cVEMP response to air conducted stimulus will be abnormal only in 20–30% (Murofushi et al.) of patients because of predominant involvement of superior vestibular nerve in acute vestibular neuritis.

In Ménière's disease, certain interesting features are observed in addition to abnormality in amplitude or absent waves and they include augmentation of VEMP in the affected ear and fluctuation of VEMP during an attack.[3]

Currently, the VEMP are more useful in the diagnosis and postoperative follow-up of various third-window syndromes including SCC dehiscence given their higher sensitivity and specificity in such clinical scenarios. In contrast, they are not much contributory in the diagnosis and follow-up of other vestibular disorders.

ELECTRONYSTAGMOGRAPHY

Electronystagmography or electrooculography is the method of recording the eye movements graphically which is essentially based on the potential difference between the retina (negative compared to cornea) and cornea which in turn is a result of the difference in the metabolism between retina and cornea. The potential difference produces an electrical dipole, which moves along with the eyes and are picked up by the electrodes placed around the eyes making either a positive or negative deflection in the graphical record depending on whether the eye moves toward or away from the particular electrode.

Procedures and Electrode Placement

Patient Preparation

Patient should be advised not to take sedative, antihistaminic drugs 48 hours prior to testing; test should be done ideally in empty stomach.

Electrode Placement

Electronystagmography is capable of recording horizontal, vertical, and torsional eye movements.

For recording horizontal eye movements, one electrode each to the right and left of the particular eye and for recording vertical eye movements one electrode above and below the eye of interest and the reference electrode has to be placed over the forehead.

Role of Nystagmography and its Interpretation

It helps us to document the presence of nystagmus, differentiate between central nystagmus or peripheral nystagmus, know the side of lesion in case of peripheral nystagmus, and know the site of lesion (probable) in case of central nystagmus.

Maneuvers to be done and results to be observed.

Initially, the presence of spontaneous nystagmus should be looked for and documented, if present. Following this, a battery of maneuver, viz., positioning, caloric stimulation, and ocular tracing has to be done sequentially, and presence of nystagmus and its various features to be observed and documented.

Spontaneous, positional, induced nystagmus points toward a vestibular pathology but ocular tracing maneuvers need not necessarily indicate a vestibular pathology always because it may be abnormal in ocular disorders too.

Advantages of this test are—it is cheap, easily available, and can be used as a permanent record to compare in future.

Disadvantage—its resolution of only one degree per second.[4,5]

Normal Electronystagmography

In case of horizontal eye movement recordings, the upward deflection is caused by movement of eyes to the right side and a downward deflection by the movement of eyes to the left side; whereas in case of vertical eye movements upward movement causes upward deflection and downward eye movement causes downward deflection; clockwise eye movements produce upward deflection and counterclockwise eye movements produce downward deflection **(Figs. 3 to 19)**.

VIDEO-OCULOGRAPHY

Video-oculography is the method of recording the eye movements with specialized cameras attached to goggles which are to be worn by the patient during the test procedure.

The cameras record the movement of the eye by keeping the center of pupil as the reference point.

There are two basic types of video-oculographic instrument namely monocular and binocular, each with its inherent advantages and disadvantages.

The essential difference between an ENG and a VOG is that ENG detects and gives a record of the eye movements based on the change in direction of the electrical dipole whereas VOG directly records the eye movements.

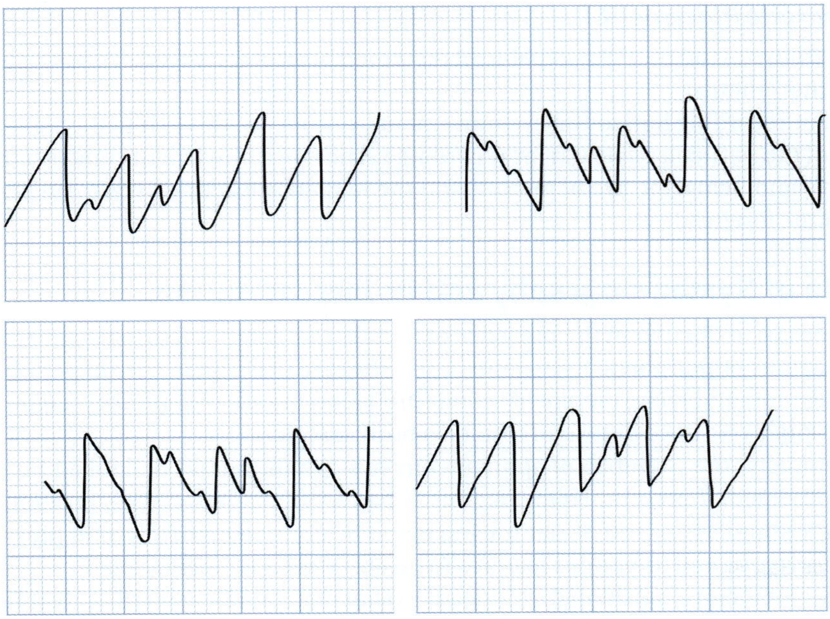

FIG. 3: Upward deflection is caused by eye movement to right side and downward deflection is caused by eye movement.

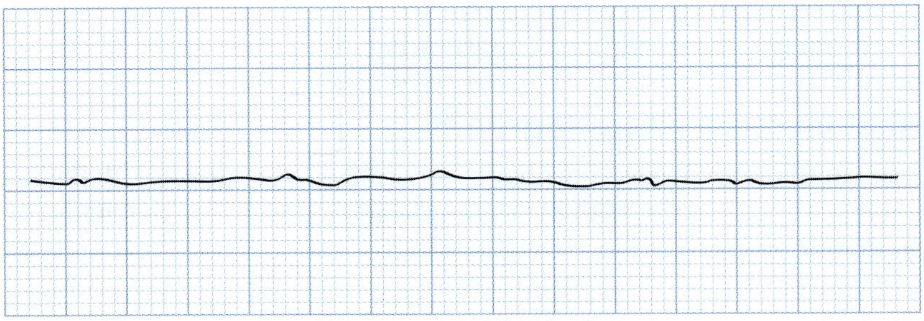

FIG. 4: Normal electronystagmography in primary gaze.

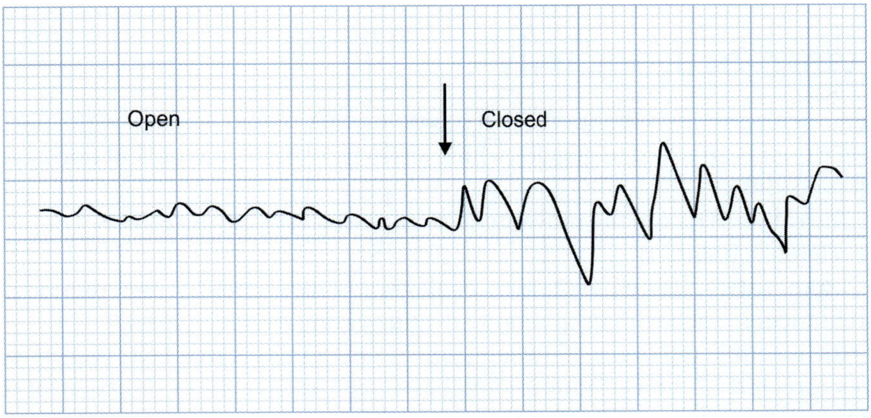

FIG. 5: Gaze evoked nystagmus—peripheral lesion (with eyes open—visual fixation present; with eyes closed—visual fixation eliminated).

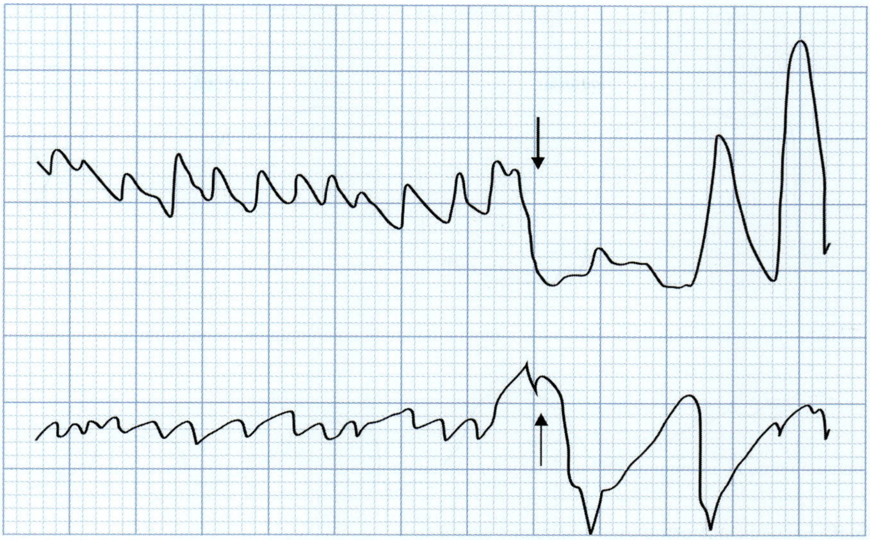

FIG. 6: Gaze evoked nystagmus—central lesion (arrows indicating eye closure).

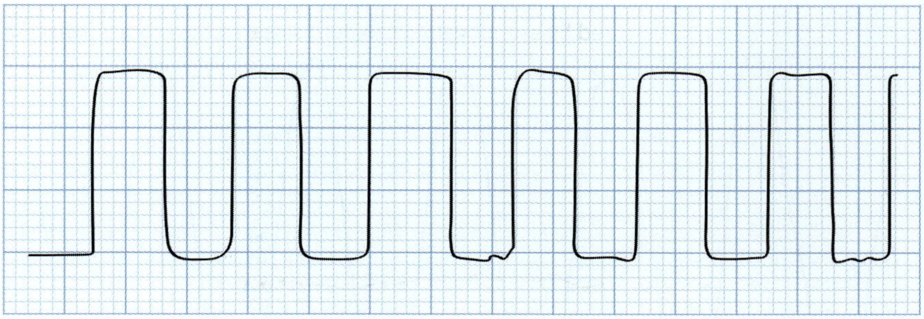

FIG. 7: Normal saccades.

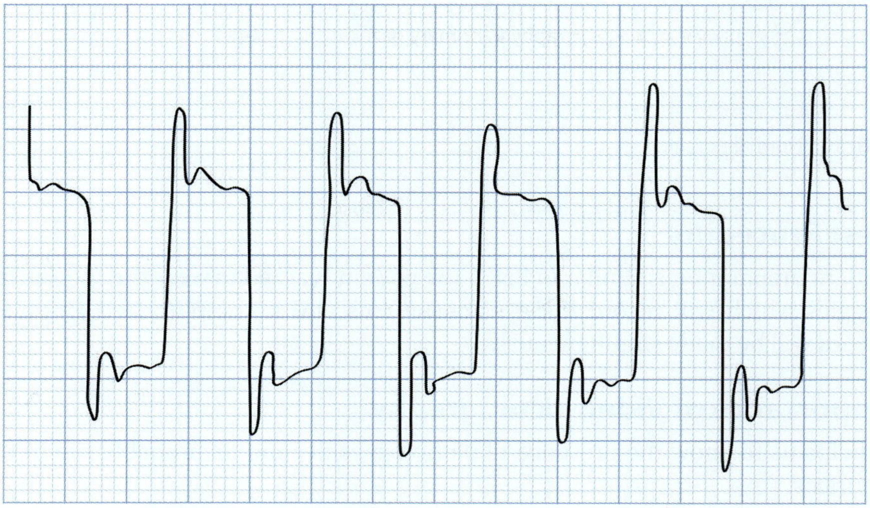

FIG. 8: Saccadic abnormalities—overshoot.

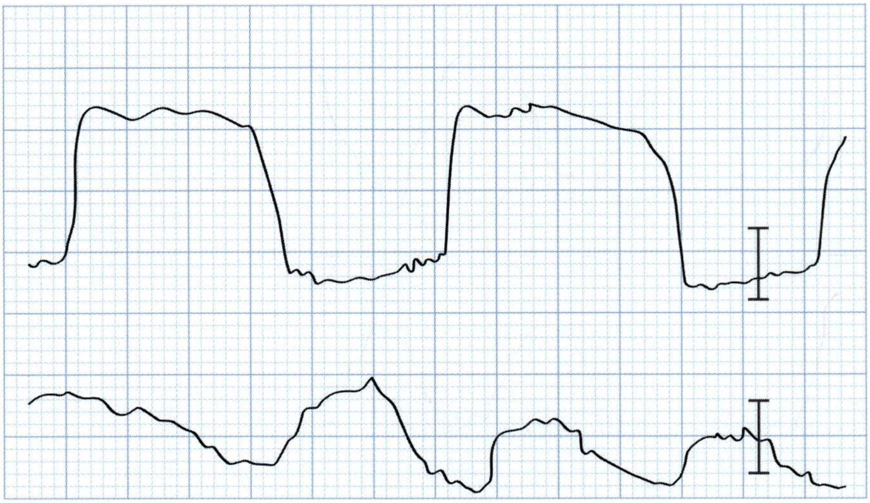

FIG. 9: Saccadic abnormalities—saccadic slowing.

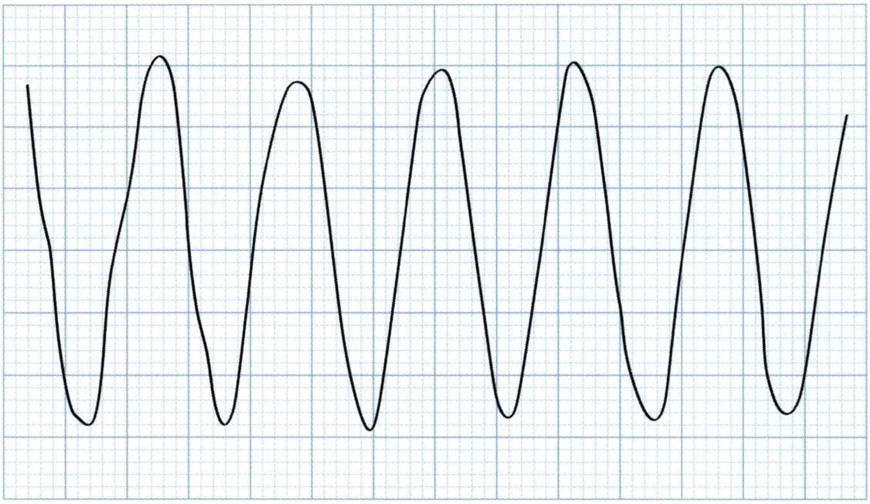

FIG. 10: Normal pursuit.

Test Procedure

Patient preparation is similar to ENG. The patient is asked to wear the specialized goggles which will record the eye movements and a computerized graphical record will be made simultaneously.

Importance of Video-oculography

It helps us to know the presence of pathology, side, and its probable site in the neuraxis.

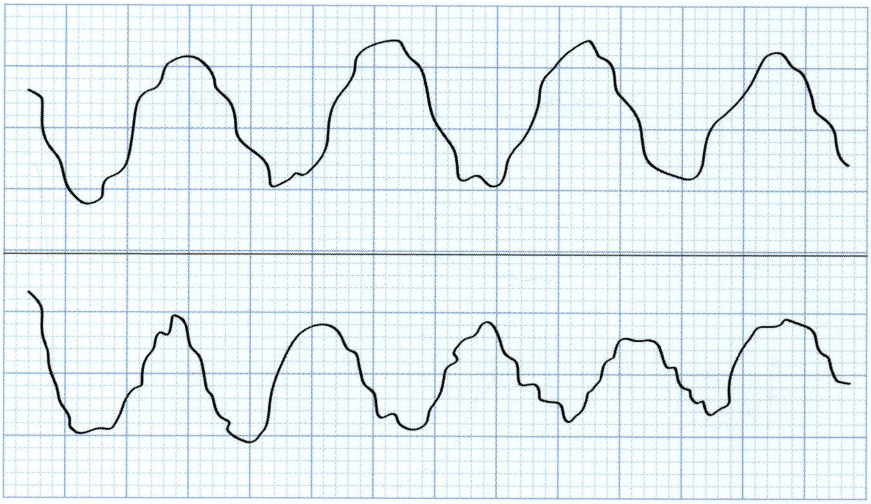

FIG. 11: Abnormal pursuit movement.

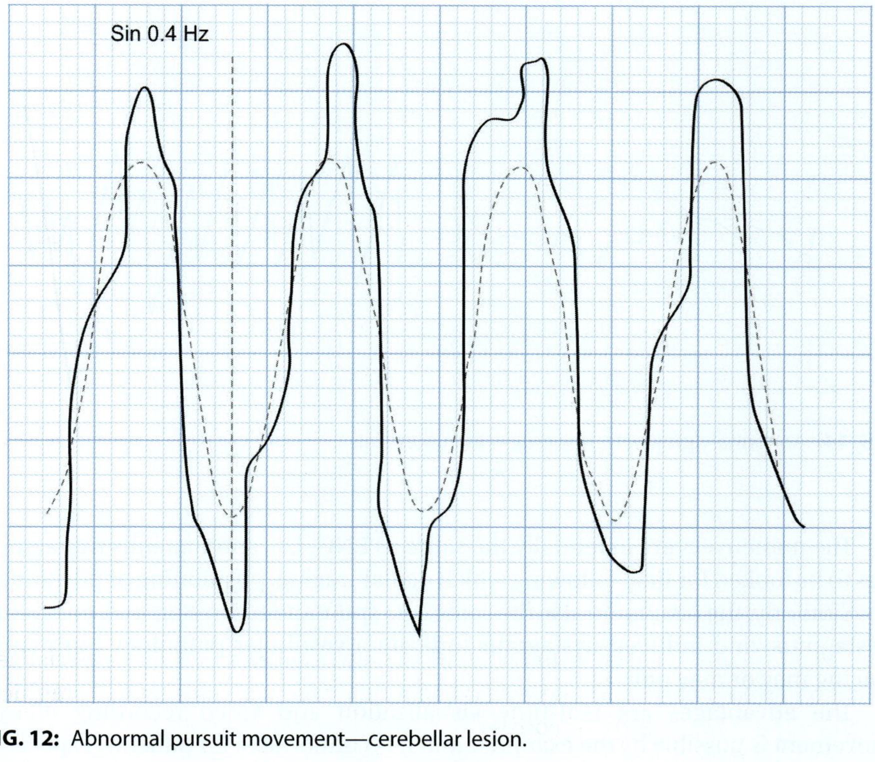

FIG. 12: Abnormal pursuit movement—cerebellar lesion.

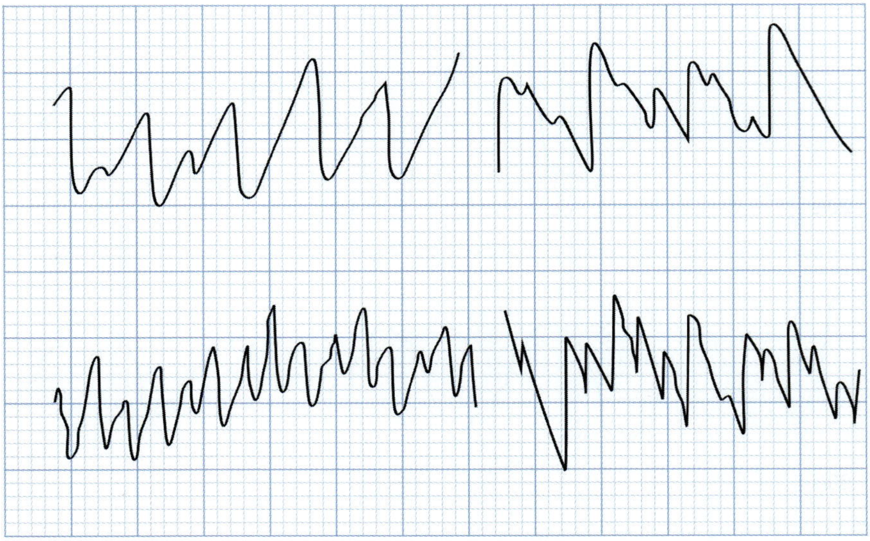

FIG. 13: Normal optokinetic response—bilaterally symmetrical.

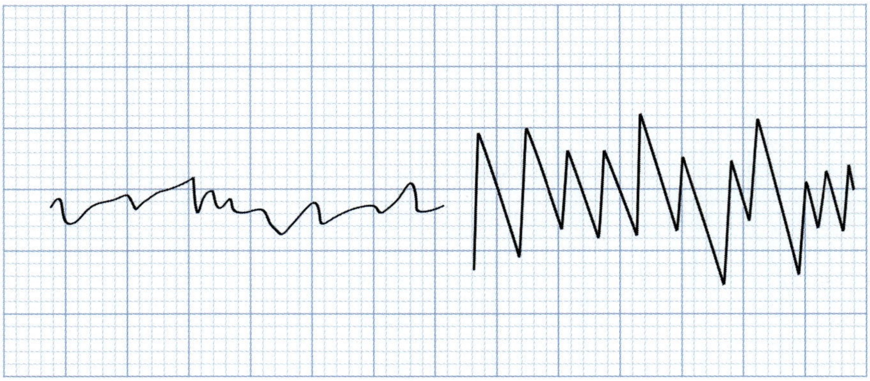

FIG. 14: Abnormal optokinetic response—asymmetrical.

The maneuvers are essentially the same as ENG, i.e., spontaneous nystagmus has to be looked for first, following which ocular tracing, positioning or positional.

Similarly, the results are also the same, i.e., spontaneous nystagmus, positional nystagmus, and induced nystagmus indicate a vestibular pathology but ocular tracing may or may not.

The advantages are real-time visualization and video recording of eye movement is possible by the examiner and it is comfortable for patients, especially children when compared to ENG. There will not be any bioelectric interference of facial muscles as seen in ENG and it is relatively quick and easy to perform since there is no need for repeated calibrations.

The main disadvantages are the cost of the instrument and it is difficult to be performed in patients with blepharoptosis.[6]

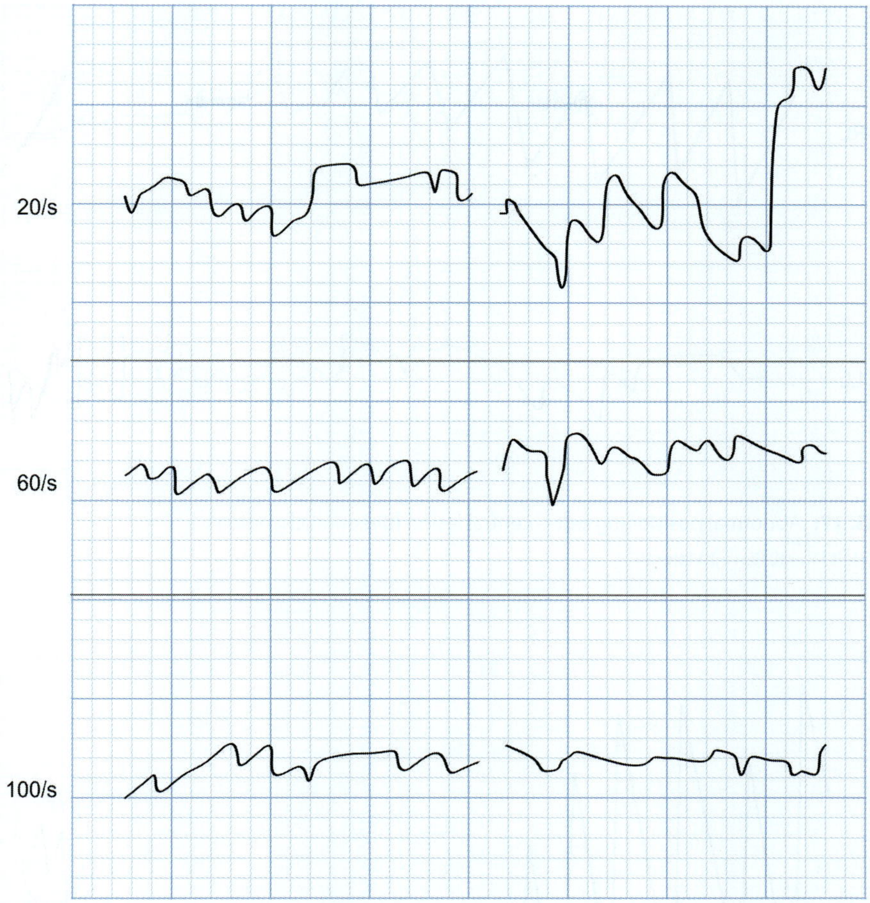

FIG. 15: Abnormal optokinetic response—declining response intensity.

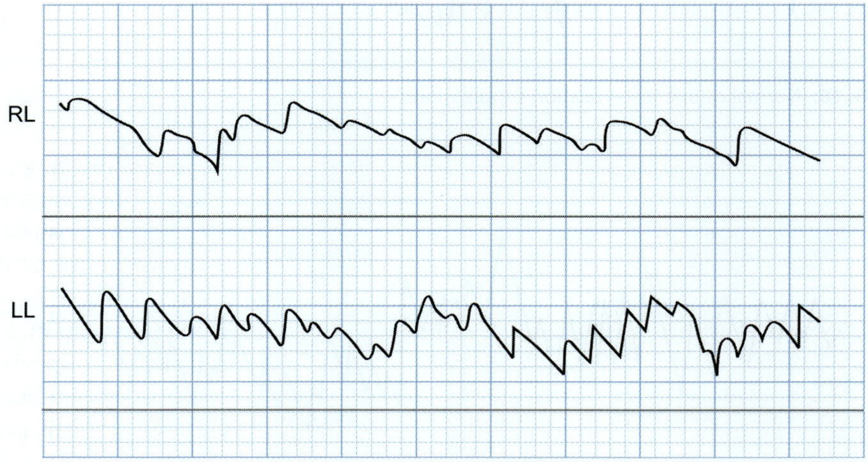

FIG. 16: Abnormal positioning test—peripheral lesion (direction is fixed).

(RL: right lateral; LL: left lateral)

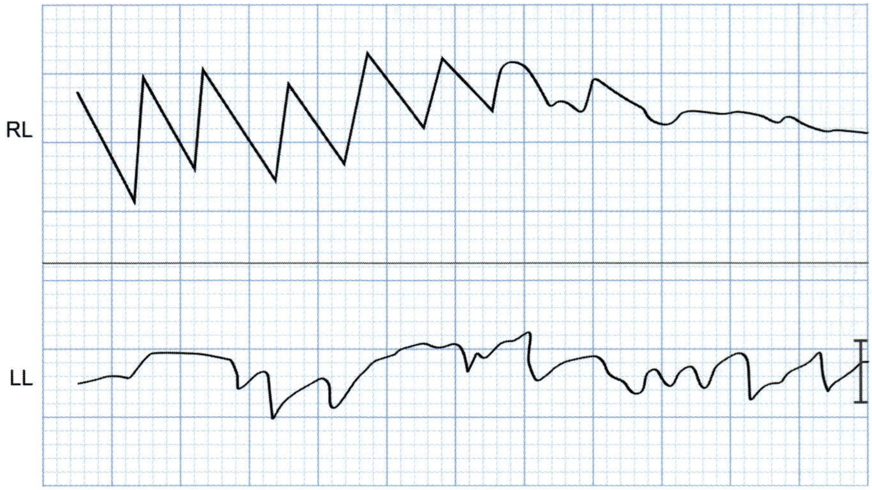

FIG. 17: Abnormal positioning test—central lesion (direction changing).
(LL: left lateral; RL: right lateral)

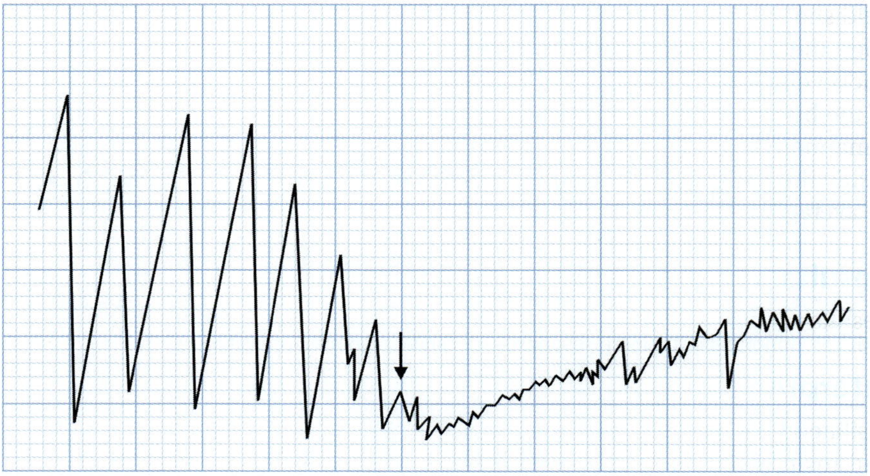

FIG. 18: Normal caloric test—fixation suppression.

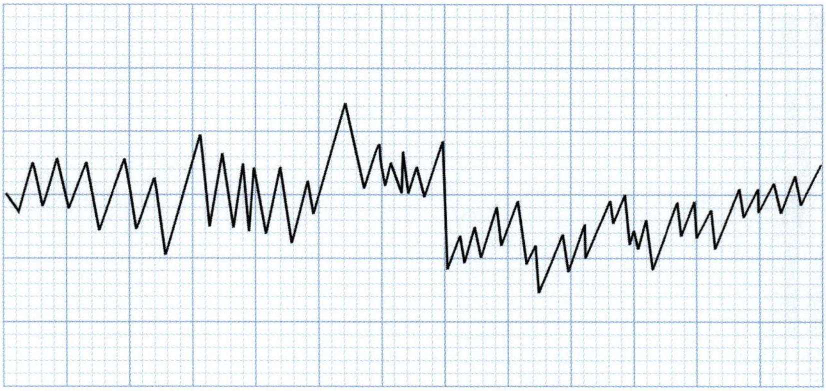

FIG. 19: Caloric test—failure of fixation suppression.

SUBJECTIVE VISUAL VERTICAL

One's ability to perceive verticality is based on the intactness of the inputs from the visual, vestibular, and somatosensory systems, and its integration and processing in the central nervous system. Various studies have shown that the contribution of the above said systems in perceiving verticality varies, and it is generally accepted that the contribution of the otolith organ is the dominant one. Eventually, disorders of otolith organs are expected to affect one's perception of verticality. Even in the absence of visual cues, normal individuals will be able to align the object with in a two degree of the true vertical. Subjective visual vertical (SVV) testing is essentially for the vestibular apparatus concerned with linear acceleration **(Fig. 20)**.

Test Procedure

There are various methods to test SVV namely bucket test and headset which uses virtual reality. The easiest among them is the bucket test which can be performed even at the bedside with simple instruments.

The patient is made to view the inside of an opaque bucket. Her/his visual field should be completely covered by the rim of the bucket. She/he is asked to align the dark line at the bottom of the bucket while the examiner rotates the bucket either to his right or left. A plumb line will be there on the outside bottom of the bucket which originates from a protractor. The protractor is fixed in such a manner so that the zero line of the protractor will coincide with the dark line inside the bucket. A total of 10 alignment trials will be made and the results will be averaged.

Results

Results can be normal or there may be ipsilateral or contralateral deviation.

Interpretation

Ipsilateral deviation of SVV is seen in acute vestibular neuritis, caudal pontine, and rostral medullary lesions whereas contralateral deviation of SVV is seen in caudal mesencephalic and rostral pontine lesions.[7-9]

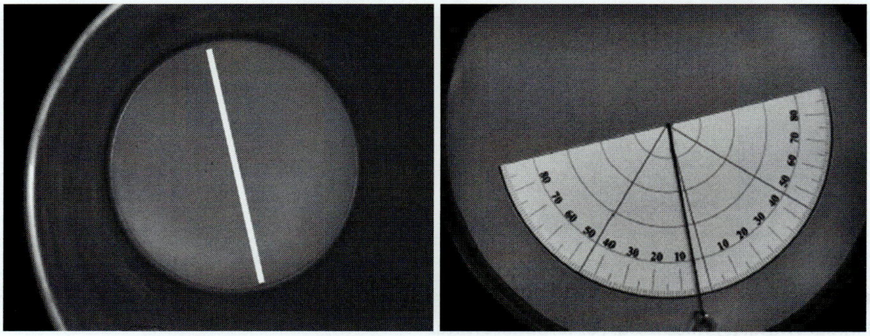

FIG. 20: Subjective visual vertical.

The deviation reverts back to normal in few weeks after the initial insult which makes them less reliable in chronic pathologies.

GAIT ANALYSIS

Gait is a complex, coordinated movement of various parts of the body that aids the human in locomotion for his various needs. To execute this task of locomotion without any difficulty we need continuous inputs from the vestibular, visual, and somatosensory systems. Hence, any vestibular disorder is expected to affect gait.

Gait Cycle

Gait cycle is shown in **Table 1** and **Figures 21A to G**.

TABLE 1: Various phases of gait cycle.

Stance phase	Swing phase
• Heel strike or initial contact • Loading response • Midstance • Terminal stance • Preswing	• Initial swing • Midswing • Terminal swing

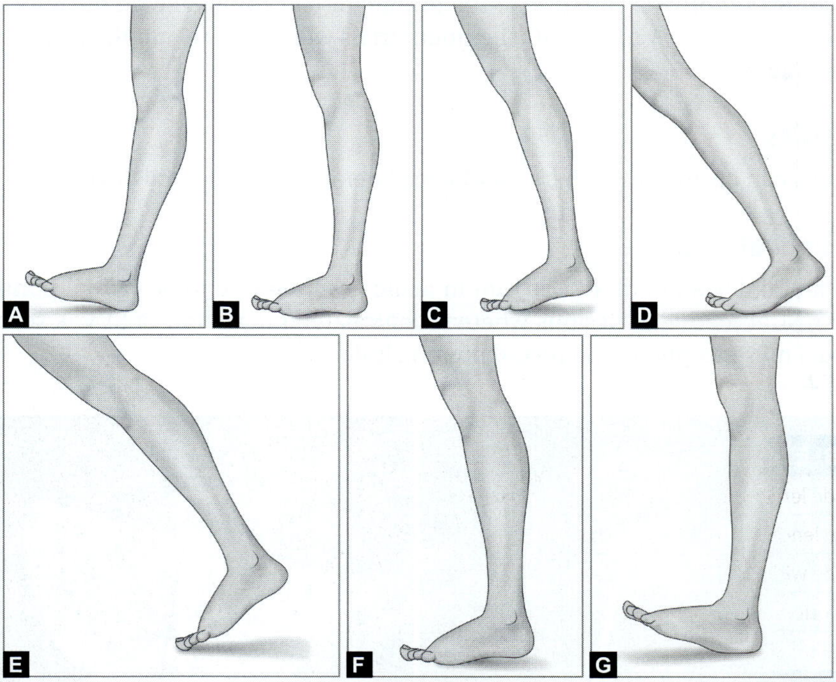

FIGS. 21A TO G: Gait cycle. (A) Loading response; (B) midstance; (C): terminal stance; (D) preswing; (E) initial swing; (F) midswing; (G) terminal swing.

Gait Parameters

It is subdivided into spatial parameters and temporal parameters **(Fig. 22)**.

- Spatial parameters **(Table 2)**
- Temporal parameters **(Table 3)**

Abnormalities of Gait Associated with Vestibular Disorders

Reduced speed, reduced stride, reduced step length, widening of step width, increased double stance time, increased stance phase, tandem walking difficulty, and steering difficulty.

Technical Aspects of Gait Analysis

The instruments available for gait analysis can be grossly classified into **(Flowchart 3)**:

- Wearable sensor-based technique is one in which the sensors are attached to various parts of the body and the sensors detect and process the signals according to the basic type of sensor used.
- Examples for sensors used in wearable system include electromyogram, accelerometers, goniometers, and magnetometers.
- As the name implies, in nonwearable based system, the sensors are not directly attached to the patient. The two subtypes of which include the image

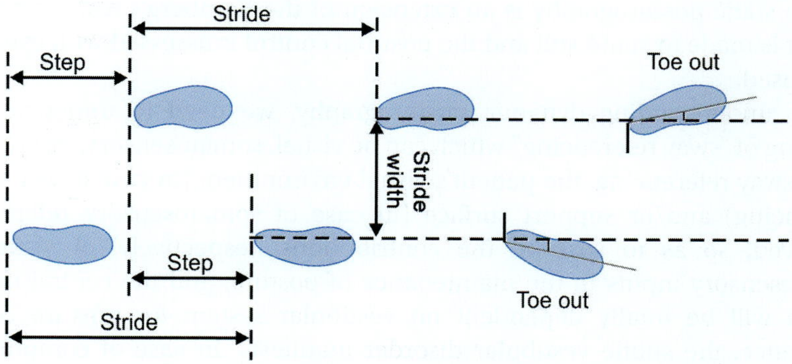

FIG. 22: Gait parameters.

TABLE 2: Spatial parameters of gait cycle.	
Stride length	Is the length between two successive steps of the same foot?
Step length	Is the length between the heel of the trailing limb to that of the leading one?
Stride width	Side-to-side distance between the two feet
Toe out	Angle between direction of progression and the reference foot line

TABLE 3: Temporal parameters of gait cycle.	
Cadence	Number of steps/unit time
Speed	Distance covered/unit time

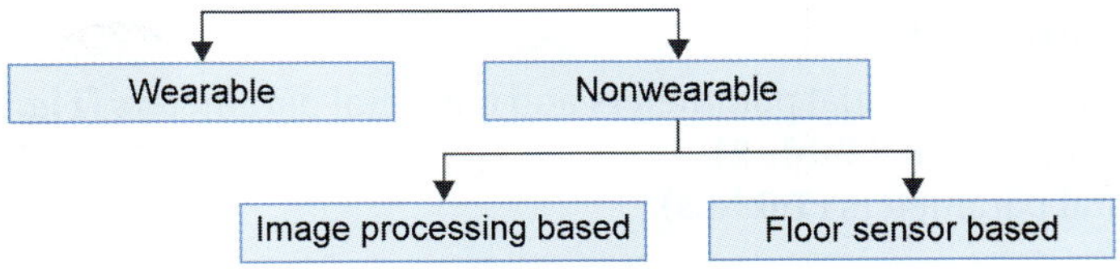

FLOWCHART 3: Technical aspects of gait analysis.

processing-based system in which images of the patient's gait will be captured and processed by specialized cameras or other optical systems and results produced whereas in the second type namely the floor sensor-based system, the gait is analyzed by the force exerted by the patient's foot on the force platforms.[7,8,10]

POSTUROGRAPHY

Posturography is the objective method of assessing one's ability of postural control. Basically, there are two types of posturography, namely, static and dynamic posturography. Static posturography is one in which the assessment of patient's postural control is done in a relatively undisturbed stance where as in dynamic posturography the assessment is done at induced disturbances of balance.

The static posturography is an extension of the Romberg's test wherein the patient is made to stand still and the postural control is assessed with eyes open and closed.

For understanding dynamic posturography, we need to understand the meaning of "sway referencing" which can be visual, somatosensory, or both.

In sway referencing, the patient's visual environment (in case of visual sway referencing) and/or support surface (in case of somatosensory referencing) is moved, so as to strip-off the contributions, respectively, of visual and somatosensory inputs in the maintenance of posture; and the central nervous system will be totally dependent on vestibular system for posture control, and hence, the subtle vestibular disorder manifests. In case of computerized dynamic posturography, the sensors detects the relative vertical force (center of mass) produced during sway underneath the heel and forefoot. The results are analyzed and produced in terms of velocity, amplitude, and frequency of sway in anteroposterior and mediolateral direction **(Fig. 23)**.[11-13]

PURE TONE AUDIOMETRY

Role of Auditory Evaluation in Patients with Vertigo

- The anatomical proximity of the auditory and the vestibular system makes them vulnerable to certain common disease which may affect them simultaneously or sequentially. For this reason, it is logical to assess auditory function in most patients with vertigo if not in all.

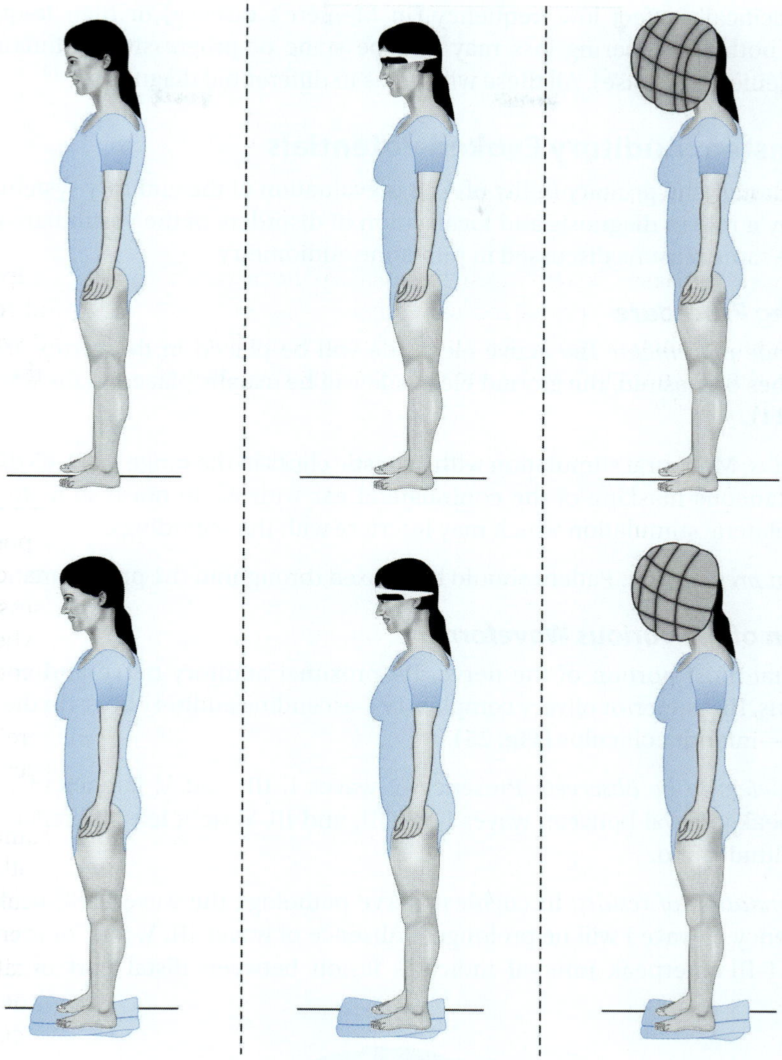

FIG. 23: Foam and dome test—visual sway referencing done with dome and somatosensory sway referencing done with foam.

- The second important contribution of hearing assessment in vertigo is to predict the reliability of a particular test in a given patient. For example, in case of VEMP when the patient's air-bone gap is greater than 20, it is not ideal to do VEMP testing by conventional tone burst stimulation.
- Few disease conditions in which vestibular system and auditory system are affected together includes otosclerosis, Ménière's disease, labyrinthitis, vestibular schwannoma, temporal bone fracture, barotraumas, Cogan's syndrome, congenital malformations, and ototoxicity.
- The pattern of hearing loss in such diseases may involve conductive apparatus, sensory neural apparatus (Ménière's disease), or both (otosclerosis). It may

specifically affect low frequency (in Ménière's disease) or high frequency or both. The hearing loss may also be static or progressive or fluctuating (Ménière's disease). All these will aid us in differential diagnosis.[12,14]

Brainstem Auditory Evoked Potentials

Even though the primary utility of ABR is evaluation of the auditory system, they do play a role in diagnosis and localization of disorders of the vestibular system for the same reasons discussed in pure tone audiometry.

Testing Procedure

Electrode placement: The active electrode will be placed in the vertex and the ear lobes or mastoid, the ground electrode will be usually placed in the forehead **(Fig. 24)**.

Stimulus: Monaural stimulation with acoustic clicks in the range of 60–65 dB with simultaneous masking of the contralateral ear with white noise so as to avoid contralateral stimulation which may interfere with the recordings.

Patient preparation: Patient should be relaxed throughout the procedure.

Origin of the Various Waveforms

I—distal most portion of the nerve, II—proximal auditory nerve and cochlear nucleus, III—superior olivary complex, IV—ascending auditory fibers in the pons, and V—inferior colliculus **(Fig. 25)**.

Parameters to be observed: Presence of waves I, III, and V, latency of I wave, interpeak interval between waves I-V, I-III, and III-V, right left difference, IV/V: I amplitude ratio.

Interpretation of results: In cochlear nerve pathology the wave I will be absent or latency of wave I will be prolonged. Absence of waves III, V, and/or increased wave I-III interpeak interval indicates lesion between distal part of the 8th

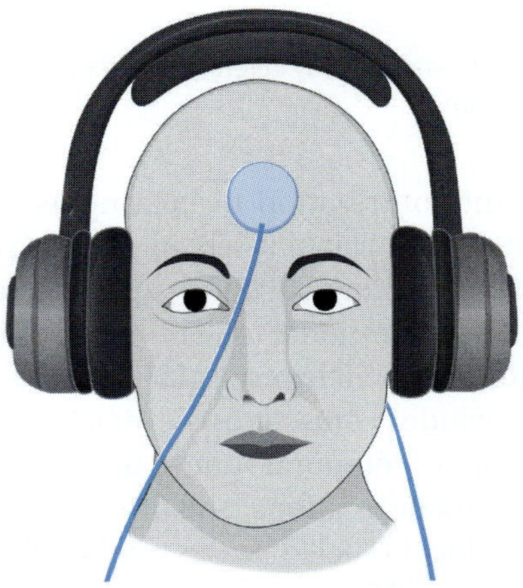

FIG. 24: Testing set-up for auditory brainstem response.

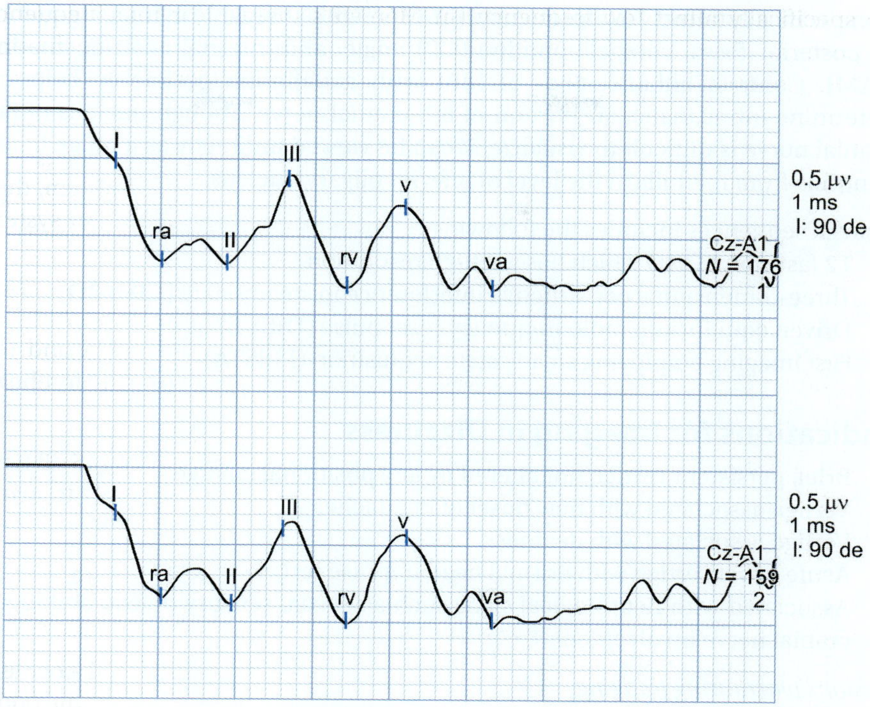

FIG. 25: Normal waveforms of auditory brainstem response.

cranial nerve and lower pons. Increased wave I–V and/or III–V interpeak interval indicates a lesion between lower pons and mesencephalon. Abnormally, *low IV/V amplitude:* I amplitude ratio points to a lesion between distal 8th nerve and mesencephalon.

LIMITATIONS

Certain components of the test are subject to variability by patient-related and nonpatient-related factors.

A normal ABR cannot exclude a brainstem lesion because a very small lesion in the brainstem, sparing the auditory pathway may not affect the ABR. Similarly, the converse is also true.[2]

TESTS FOR STRUCTURAL INTEGRITY OF VESTIBULAR SYSTEM-NEUROIMAGING

Imaging in vertigo is very important to rule out central causes and also to detect treatable peripheral causes of dizziness. There are many available modalities for visualizing vestibular apparatus, temporal bone, and posterior cranial fossa structures. It includes computed tomography (CT) brain, magnetic resonance imaging (MRI) brain, and its various sequences. CT brain is a beneficial modality to rule out structural lesions though accurate diagnosis is difficult. CT temporal bone scan is extremely useful in viewing SCCs. MRI is valuable in imaging lesions in posterior fossa, cerebellopontine (CP) angle, and internal acoustic meatus (IAM). Contrast enhancement of MRI with gadolinium preferably helps to determine intracanalicular portion of 8th cranial nerve. Though nucleus of 8th cranial nerve is difficult to visualize, it can be viewed indirectly as a bulge in 4th ventricle from medulla at the level of inferior olivary nucleus.[15]

Special sequences includes the following:
- T2 fast spin ECHO which has got high resolution
- Three-dimensional constructive interference in steady state (CISS-3D)
- Driven equilibrium radio frequency reset pulse (DRIVE)
- Fast imaging employing steady state acquisition (FIESTA)

Indications for Imaging in Dizziness

- Brief, persistent vertigo not altered by any positional change.
- Vertigo associated with new onset of headache.
- Vertigo associated with deafness.
- Acute onset vertigo with normal head impulse test.
- Associated with neurological signs such as ataxia, sensory defect, and lower cranial nerve involvement.[16]

Lesions warranting imaging:
- *Peripheral causes*:
  - *Labyrinthine lesions:* Labyrinthitis, Ménière's disease, perilymphatic fistula, semicircular canal dehiscence, labyrinthine trauma, and otosclerosis.
  - *Temporal bone lesions:* Cholesterol granuloma, cholesteatoma, temporal bone fractures, and tumors.[17]
- *Central causes*:
  - Acoustic neuroma, vascular lesions of brainstem, and posterior fossa, demyelinating disorders, brainstem malignancy, and basilar migraine.[17]

Labyrinthine Lesions

Membranous Labyrinth

Labyrinthitis is an inflammation of membranous labyrinth. MRI shows contrast enhancement in acute phase, high signal enhancement in T2 Flair, high signal intensity than cerebrospinal fluid (CSF) in T1, and low signal intensity than CSF in T2 weighted image (T2WI).

Bony Labyrinth

Trauma to temporal bone is associated with injury to bony labyrinth thereby resulting in perilymphatic fistula. The defect in this condition is seen in round window, oval window, or otic capsule. CT of temporal bone with at least 1 mm resolution is useful to identify this defect. Axial image of CT might show air pockets within vestibule due to fistula (pneumolabyrinth). MRI, though not as useful as CT in imaging bone is however useful in picking up tumors and multiple sclerosis plaques which causes the defect. Precontrast T1 weighted image (T1WI) shows high signal intensity due to methemoglobin in hemorrhage following trauma. Axial contrast enhanced T1WI shows enhancement in basal turn of cochlea.[18]

Canal Dehiscence

Canal dehiscence is associated with vertigo and oscillopsia. It results from defect in the bone overlying SCC thereby resulting in abnormal fluid mechanics of middle ear. Coronal image reformatted from transverse multidetector row CT images of temporal bone shows the defect in the canal. MRI T2 and fast spin echo shows clear connection between inner ear and brain fluid.[18]

Congenital Malformation of Labyrinth

It is mostly associated with dilation of vestibular aqueduct. It is diagnosed in MRI with diameter at midpoint of aqueduct >1 mm and diameter at the opercular origin >2 mm.

Labyrinthitis Ossificans

Suppurative bacterial infection from meningeal spread results in sclerosing type of labyrinthitis, which results in ossification of cochlea from the basal turn to apex. CT imaging is best modality in this condition. Early CT scan shows ill-defined haziness in labyrinth while late stage scan shows total white out of labyrinth. T2WI/fast spin echo shows loss of normal signal intensity of fluid in the labyrinth.

Differentiation of it from congenital otic dysplasia is made by maintained contour of otic capsule. Fibro-osseous replacement of cochlea is of paramount importance, when cochlear implantation is contemplated.[1]

Otosclerosis

Otosclerosis is associated with idiopathic infiltrative process of petrous temporal bone. CT imaging is more sensitive.

In early stages of otosclerosis, a radiolucent focus may be seen at the fissula ante fenestram, which is a cleft of fibrocartilaginous tissue located just anterior to the oval window. As the disease progresses, this lucency involves the margins of the oval and round windows and may even produce multiple radiolucent foci. Extension of the disease to the otic capsule may produce imaging signs of both fenestral and cochlear otosclerosis in the same patient. Cochlear otosclerosis is characterized by low-attenuation foci around the basal turn of the cochlea, though some lesions may also involve the lateral walls of the internal auditory canal (IAC) and the cochlear promontory.

In severe otosclerosis, a low attenuation ring sometimes surrounds the cochlea, known as the *double-ring sign*. In the later healing phase, CT may show a “heaped-up” appearance along the margins of the oval and round windows and around the cochlea, indicating new bone formation.

Ménière’s Disease (Idiopathic Endolymphatic Hydrops)

In Ménière’s disease 3D fluid-attenuated inversion recovery (FLAIR) MRI is more sensitive. It clearly delineates the perilymphatic and endolymphatic spaces of inner ear after intratympanic injection of gadolinium diethylenetriaminepentaacetic acid (DTPA). Ideally time interval of 24 hours is required between contrast administration and MRI. Vestibular enhancement is observed first, followed by advance of the enhancement to the basal cochlear turn and semicircular canals, and finally, the apical turn of the cochlea.

Petrous Temporal Bone Lesions

The petrous apex lesions cause dizziness owing to its relation to IAM and orifice of vestibular aqueduct to the posterosuperior surface or cerebellar aspect of petrous bone. Air cells from middle ear cleft also invade the petrous apex through various tracts.

Cholesterol Granuloma

More commonly seen in patients with pneumatized petrous apex and long-standing otitis media. These lesions are typically viewed in CT as isointense expansile lesion with smooth border and in MRI as hyperintense nonenhancing expansile lesions.[18]

Cholesteatoma

Petrous apex cholesteatoma and epidermoids account for 4–9% of petrous apex lesions. Congenital types of cholesteatoma are more common. CT shows nonenhancing expansile lesions at petrous apex very similar to cholesterol granuloma, the only differentiating feature being the presence of varying degrees of bone destruction. T1WI of MRI shows intermediate-to-low signal intensity. T2WI/FLAIR presents high signal intensity without enhancement and diffusion restriction in diffusion weighted imaging (DWI).[18]

Temporal Bone Fractures

It follows cranial and cervical trauma. Though all pattern of injury might cause temporal fracture, dizziness is more common with transverse type fractures which damages the nerve in the inner ear. Imaging modality of choice is head CT with petrous temporal bone fine slice multiplanar bone window reformats. It is mostly associated with blow to occipital bone and labyrinthine capsule too. About 50% of patients show pneumotympanum.[18]

Tumors

Tumors of petrous temporal bone associated with dizziness which necessitate imaging includes meningioma, paraganglioma, chondrosarcomas, metastasis, nasopharyngeal carcinoma, and petrous internal carotid artery (ICA) aneurysm.

Vestibular Nerve

Acoustic Schwannoma

It is the most common tumor associated with the nerve. It takes origin from IAM and extends into CP angle. It is present as a solid nodular mass in intracanalicular portion of the nerve. This widening of the canal results in trumpeted IAM sign. Extra canalicular extension of the mass into CP angle causes ice cream cone appearance. Smaller masses are solid while larger ones shows cystic degeneration.

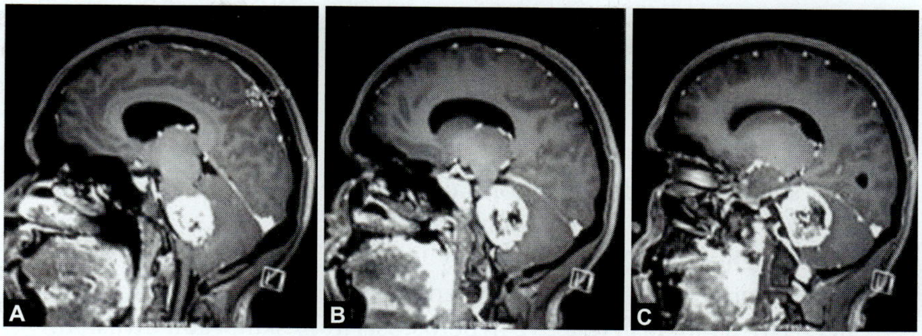

FIGS. 26A TO C: T1 postcontrast sagittal sections showing contrast enhancing lesion in cerebellopontine angle.

CT shows erosion and widening of IAC with contrast enhancement. T1WI of MRI presents with hypodense cystic lesions, T2WI with heterogenous hyperintense lesions. These lesions enhance with gadolinium **(Figs. 26A to C)**.

Vestibular Neuronitis

Patients present with acute onset dizziness. On high field strength 3T MRI with gadolinium contrast isolated enhancement of nerve in the inner ear is visualized. This suggests viral or inflammatory cause.

Vascular Lesions of Internal Auditory Canal

This condition presents with acute onset of vertigo and deafness and may follow infarction of labyrinthine artery. But isolated involvement of labyrinthine artery is rare. It is usually associated with involvement of vertebrobasilar system. When associated with cerebellar or brainstem signs it mainly results from infarction of anterior inferior cerebellar artery. MRI with MR angiography is indicated in this condition.

Cerebellopontine Angle Lesion

Most common pathology associated with CP angle lesions include neoplasm:

- *Neoplastic lesions*:
  - Acoustic neuroma
  - Meningioma
  - Epidermoid cyst
  - Hemangioma
  - Metastasis
- *Non-neoplastic lesions*:
  - Meningitis
  - Traumatic
  - Demyelinating
  - Siderosis
  - Sarcoidosis
- *Meningioma:* Meningioma is the most common type of extra-axial neoplasm and accounts for 14–20% of intracranial neoplasms. It is a nonglial neoplasm that originates from the arachnoid cap cells of the meninges.

- *Plain film skull*:
  - Enlarged meningeal artery grooves
  - Hyperostosis or lytic regions
  - Calcification
- *CT brain*:
  - 60% slightly hyperdense to normal brain.
  - 20–30% have some calcification.
  - 72% brightly and homogenously contrast enhance, less frequent in malignant or cystic variants, hyperostosis is typical in meningiomas and needs to distinguish reactive hyperostosis from skull vault invasion.
- *MRI brain*:
  - On T1WI hypo- to isointense compared to gray matter.
  - *On T2WI hypo- to iso- to hyperintense to gray matter (the intensity varies according to tumoral cellularity:* Higher the cellularity, lower the signal intensity on both TI and T2WI) (most common extra-axial type of tumor, following acoustic neuroma. CT shows iso to hyperdense lesions with calcifications. T1WI and T2WI MRI show variable intensity depending on tumor cellularity. Tumor with high cellularity shows low signal intensity. Enhances homogenously with contrast. It also shows restriction in DWI. Angiography presents with dense venous filling and spoke wheel appearance. It shows the characteristic dural tail in imaging.
- *Specific signs*:
  - CSF cleft sign (the cleft was regarded as representing a thin rim of CSF between tumor and brain parenchyma).
  - Dural tail (as a result of thickening of the dura).
- *Angiography*:
  - *"Mother-in-law sign":* "Comes early, stays late, very dense"—tumor blush.

Meningiomas have dual blood supply from both pial vessels, i.e., ICA supplies periphery of the tumor and meningeal vessels, i.e., external carotid artery (ECA) supplies core of the tumor. They typically show a spoke-wheel appearance and dense venous filling.

Brainstem and Cerebellar Lesions

It is due to the involvement of the vestibular nuclei and the corresponding tracts.

- Infections—meningitis, epidural abscess, and encephalitis
- Posterior circulation strokes
- Structural—hydrocephalus
- Demyelinating—multiple sclerosis
- Brainstem tumors

The CT and MRI are invaluable in the evaluation of infections, vascular malformations, ischemic lesions, structural lesions, brainstem tumors, and demyelinating lesions in the brainstem and cerebellum **(Figs. 27A and B)**.

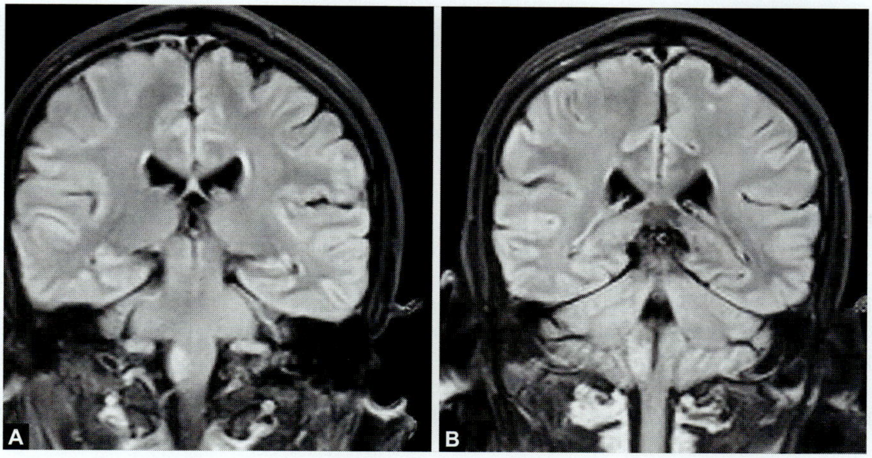

FIGS. 27A AND B: T2 fluid-attenuated inversion recovery coronal images showing hyperintense lesion in the left lateral half of medulla.

CONCLUSION

The management of dizzy patients depends upon understanding of the contribution of vestibular system in its causation. This can be accomplished by a clinical evaluation which in turn can be assisted by laboratory investigations and neuroimaging in selected patients. These laboratory investigations play useful role in localizing the lesion, to arrive at a probable etiology, and also to know the severity of the disease in many instances. Hence, a basic understanding about the principle of each tests, test procedure, result interpretation, role in specific diseases, and their advantages and disadvantages are essential to select the appropriate test in a given clinical context because, inappropriate tests or multiple tests may be a cost constraint and also leads to unnecessary confusion in sorting out a management plan.

REFERENCES

1. Bisdorff A, Von Brevern M, Lempert T, Newman-Toker DE. Classification of vestibular symptoms: towards an international classification of vestibular disorders. J Vestib Res. 2009;19(1-2):1-3.
2. Aminoff MJ. Aminoff's Electrodiagnosis in Clinical Neurology, 6th edition. Philadelphia, US: Saunders, Elsevier Health Sciences; 2012.
3. Rosengren SM, Welgampola MS, Colebatch JG. Vestibular evoked myogenic potentials: past, present and future. Clinical Neurophysiol. 2010;121(5):636-51.
4. Farkashidy J. Electronystagmography: Its clinical application. Can Med Assoc J. 1966;94(8):368.
5. Rubin W. Electronystagmography: a review of 17 years experience. Ann Otol Rhinol Laryngol. 1975;84(4 Pt 1):541-3.

6. Gans RE. Video-oculography: A new diagnostic technology for vestibular patients. The Hearing Journal. 2001;54(5):40-2.
7. Brandt T, Dieterich M, Strupp M. Vertigo and dizziness. London: Springer-Verlag London Limited; 2005.
8. Brandt T. Vertigo: Its Multisensory Syndromes. Berlin, Germany: Springer Science & Business Media; 2013.
9. Howard IP, Hu G. Visually induced reorientation illusions. Perception. 2001;30(5):583-600.
10. Muro-de-la-Herran A, Garcia-Zapirain B, Mendez-Zorrilla A. Gait analysis methods: an overview of wearable and non-wearable systems, highlighting clinical applications. Sensors (Basel). 2014;14(2):3362-94.
11. Baloh RW, Jacobson KM, Beykirch K, Honrubia V. Static and dynamic posturography in patients with vestibular and cerebellar lesions. Arch Neurol. 1998;55(5):649-54.
12. McGarry GW. In Gleeson M (Ed). Scott-Brown's Otorhinolaryngology: Head and Neck Surgery, 7th edition. London: Hodder Arnold Publication; 2008.
13. Visser JE, Carpenter MG, van der Kooij H, Bloem BR. The clinical utility of posturography. Clin Neurophysiol. 2008;119(11):2424-36.
14. Ruckenstein MJ. Vertigo and dysequilibrium with associated hearing loss. Otolaryngologic Clinics of North America. 2000;33(3):535-62.
15. Bronstein A. In: Bronstein A (Ed). Oxford Textbook of Vertigo and Imbalance. Oxford, UK: Oxford University Press; 2013.
16. Wippold FJ, Turski PA. Vertigo and hearing loss. Am J Neuroradiology. 2009;30(8):1623-5.
17. Patkar D, Yevankar G, Parikh R. Radiology in Vertigo and Dizziness. Int J Otorhinolaryngol Clin. 2012;4(2):86-92.
18. Park MK, Kim KM, Lee N, Jung HH, Chae SW. The usefulness of magnetic resonance imaging for acute isolated vertigo patients in the emergency department. [online] Available from www.advancedotology.org/sayilar/83/buyuk/162-166.pdf. [Last accessed April, 2025].

6 CHAPTER

International Classification of Vestibular Disorders

Venkatesh Perumalsamy, Dulari Gupta, Avinash Alashetty, Sarala G

ABSTRACT

This chapter discusses the need for the classification of vestibular disorders and the structure and pattern of classification. It focuses on the clinical categorization of primary and secondary vestibular symptoms. The international classification of vestibular disorders (ICVD) is divided into four layers. Layer I consists of symptoms and signs—primary vestibular vertigo and dizziness are described. Layer II includes clinical syndromes—this brings together the signs with the disorders causing them. Layer III-A—names the diseases and disorders and layer III-B focuses on the pathophysiologic mechanisms (pathoanatomic, pathophysiologic, and etiologic mechanisms) underlying vestibular disorders.

INTRODUCTION

Classifications and definitions are essential for explicit communication between clinicians and researchers. Definite diagnostic criteria are required for research purposes, for epidemiological studies as well as for diagnosis and treatment of patients. Disease definitions are fundamental for professional communication in clinical practice, research, and public health settings. Diagnostic criteria are of paramount importance in diseases that do not have any pathognomonic diagnostic tests (e.g., migraine). They are equally important in diseases where there is an overlap of signs and symptoms despite having supportive laboratory tests like in the diagnosis of vestibular disorders.

SCOPE FOR THE INTERNATIONAL CLASSIFICATION OF VESTIBULAR DISORDERS INITIATIVE

The definition of vestibular symptoms and classification of vestibular disorders is the major objective of the international classification of vestibular disorders (ICVD).[1] Acceptance of the classification throughout the world and cautious usage of the same is the next most important thing. Barany's vestibular society is actively seeking inputs from various neurology forums and otorhinolaryngology associations across the world for a better classification of vestibular disorders **(Flowchart 1 and Table 1)**.[2,3]

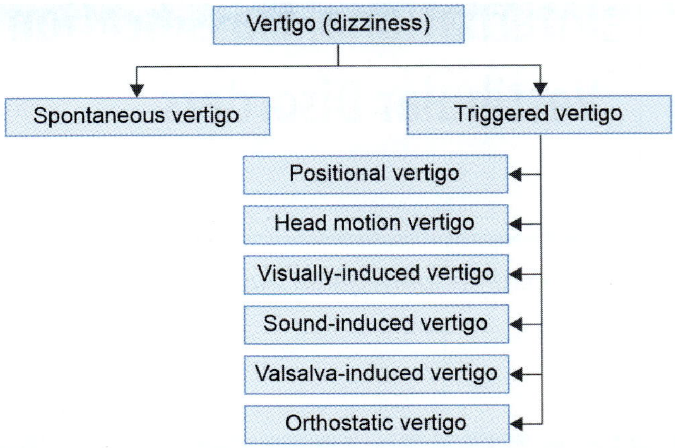

FLOWCHART 1: Classification of vertigo.

TABLE 1: Definition of vestibular symptoms.

Dizziness	Sensation of disturbed or impaired spatial orientation without a false or distorted sense of motion
Vertigo	Sensation of self-motion (of head/body) when no self-motion is occurring or the sensation of distorted self-motion during an otherwise normal head movement
Vestibulovisual symptoms **(Table 2)**	Visual symptoms usually result from vestibular pathology or the interplay between visual and vestibular systems. These include false sensations of motion or tilting of the visual surround and visual distortion (blur) linked to vestibular (rather than optical) failure
Postural symptoms **(Table 3)**	Balance symptoms related to maintenance of postural stability, occurring only while upright (seated, standing, or walking)

TABLE 2: Description of vestibulovisual symptoms.

Vestibulovisual symptoms	**Description**
External vertigo	False sensation that the visual surrounding is spinning or flowing
Oscillopsia	False sensation that the visual surrounding is oscillating
Visual lag	False sensation that the visual surround follows behind a head movement with a delay or makes a brief drift after the head movement is completed
Visual tilt	False perception of the visual surround as oriented off the true vertical
Movement-induced blur	Reduced visual acuity during or momentarily after a head movement

The ICVD plans to include all the disorders arising from the vestibular cortex to the inner ear including vestibulocerebellar brainstem connections. In addition to this, other illnesses where vestibular symptoms are more prominent are also

TABLE 3: Description of postural symptoms.	
Postural symptoms	**Description**
Unsteadiness	Feeling of being unstable while seated, standing, or walking without a particular directional preference
Directional pulsion	Feeling of being unstable with a tendency to veer or fall in a particular direction while seated, standing, or walking
A balance-related near-fall	Sensation of imminent fall (without a completed fall) related to strong unsteadiness, directional pulsion, or other vestibular symptoms (e.g., vertigo)
A balance-related fall	Completed fall related to strong unsteadiness, directional pulsion, or other vestibular symptom (e.g., vertigo)

going to be considered significant. The goal of the ICVD initiative was to develop a comprehensive classification scheme and definitions of individual vestibular disease disorders that would be acceptable worldwide.

Work on the ICVD began in 2006 under the aegis of the Classification Committee of Barany Society (CCBS). Subcommittees were set up to outline definitions and diagnostic criteria for primary vestibular disorders. Each subcommittee was headed by a member of the Barany Society with at least members from three continents; including at least one clinical neurologist and one otolaryngologist. These definitions were presented in the biennials of the published Journal of Vestibular Research.

DEFINITION OF SECONDARY VESTIBULAR SYMPTOMS

- *Spontaneous vertigo (or dizziness)*: Vertigo (or dizziness) that occurs without an obvious trigger.
- *Triggered vertigo (or dizziness)*: Vertigo (or dizziness) that occurs with an obvious trigger.
- *Positional vertigo (or dizziness)*: Vertigo (or dizziness) triggered by and occurring after a change in head position in space relative to gravity.
- *Head motion vertigo (or dizziness)*: Vertigo (or dizziness) occurs only during head motion (i.e., time-locked to the head movement).
- *Visually-induced vertigo (or dizziness)*: Vertigo (or dizziness) triggered by a complex, distorted, large field, or moving visual stimulus, including the relative motion of the visual surrounding associated with body movements.
- *Sound-induced vertigo (or dizziness)*: Vertigo (or dizziness) triggered by an auditory stimulus.
- *Valsalva-induced vertigo (or dizziness)*: Vertigo (or dizziness) triggered by any bodily maneuver that tends to increase intracranial or middle ear pressure.
- *Orthostatic vertigo (or dizziness)*: Vertigo (or dizziness) triggered by and occurring on arising (i.e., a change of body posture from lying to sitting or sitting to standing).

INTERNATIONAL CLASSIFICATION OF VESTIBULAR DISORDERS STRUCTURE

The proposed structure of the ICVD includes four layers as shown in **Flowcharts 2 and 3.**[1]

International Classification of Vestibular Disorders Layer I: Symptoms and Signs

Four cardinal vestibular symptoms:

1. Vertigo
2. Dizziness

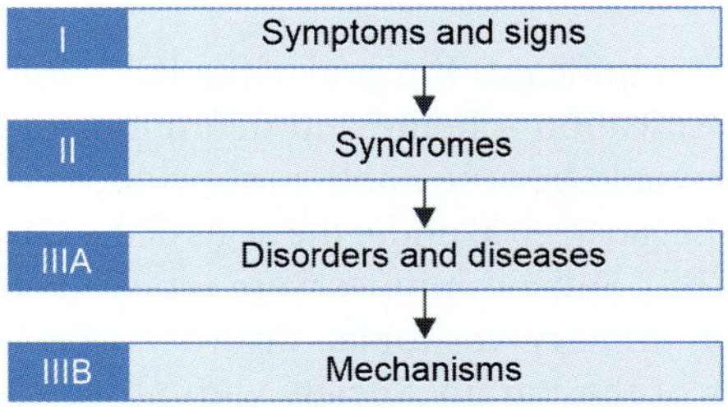

FLOWCHART 2: Four-layer framework of the international classification of vestibular disorders.

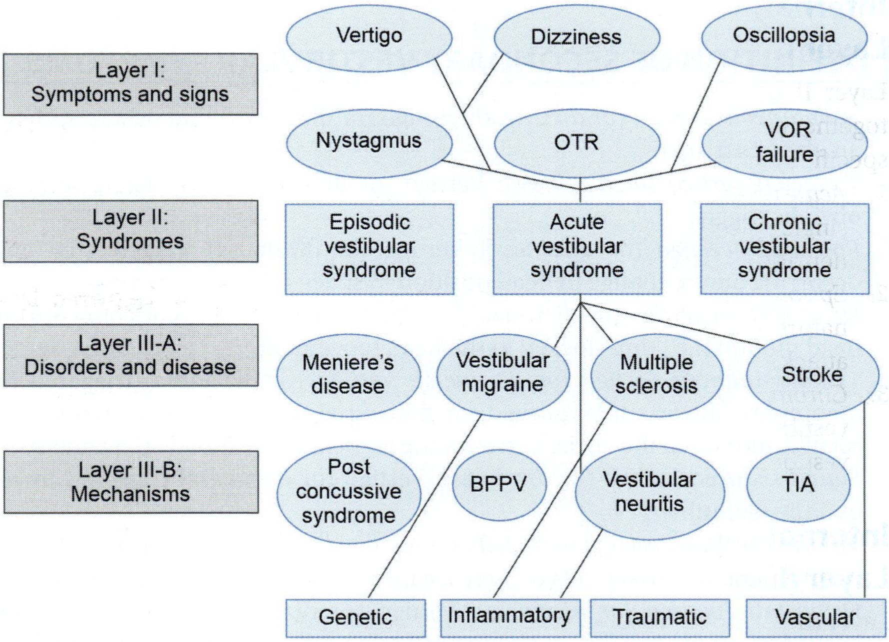

FLOWCHART 3: Schematic representation of three layers of the international classification of vestibular disorders classification.

(BPPV: benign paroxysmal positional vertigo; OTR: ocular tilt reaction; TIA: transient ischemic attack; VOR: vestibular ocular reflex)

3. Vestibulovisual symptoms
4. Postural symptoms.

This layer was defined first since all other layers are based on the outcomes of combinations of signs and symptoms defined in this layer. Only the four primary vestibular symptoms of vertigo, dizziness, vestibulovisual symptoms, and postural symptoms have been considered. Secondary symptoms such as nausea, vomiting, and anxiety have not been included. The symptoms were defined according to the following rules:

- Be nonoverlapping and nonhierarchical. Thus, one or more symptoms can coexist in patients.
- No "vestibular" symptom had a totally specific meaning in terms of topology or nosology and its pathogenesis was likely to be incompletely understood.
- Symptom definitions should be purely phenomenological, without reference to any specific theory on pathogenesis.

The new classification distinguishes vertigo (a false sense of motion of spinning or nonspinning quality) and dizziness (disturbed spatial orientation without a false sense of motion). Vertigo and dizziness are each divided into two categories, spontaneous and triggered. Vestibulovisual symptoms have been classified separately since vestibular disease presents with many different visual manifestations. Symptoms occurring on change of posture have been named "unsteadiness" over the older ambiguous terms of "imbalance" or "disequilibrium."

International Classification of Vestibular Disorders Layer II: Syndromes

Layer II offers an intermediate layer of syndromic classification that brings together symptoms and signs with the diseases or disorders causing them. Three specific syndromes have been elucidated:

1. *Acute vestibular syndrome*: Diseases and disorders that usually manifest with a single episode of sudden onset vestibular symptoms and signs (e.g., vestibular neuritis or acute stroke).
2. *Episodic vestibular syndrome*: Diseases and disorders that are recurrent by nature (e.g., Meniere's disease, vestibular migraine, or transient ischemic attack).
3. *Chronic vestibular syndrome*: Diseases and disorders that produce persistent vestibular symptoms and signs over an extended period of time (bilateral vestibular failure or cerebellar degeneration).

International Classification of Vestibular Disorders Layer III-A: Disorders and Diseases

Layer III-A describes vestibular diseases and disorders. The ICVD will use existing terms for vestibular disorders and diseases wherever possible. New terms will be developed only for conditions not included in previous classifications. If many existing terms are used to define the same disease entity, the ICVD will choose the most appropriate term for its classification. In the diagnosis of most vestibular

diseases, there is no single pathognomonic test or clinical finding. Thus, most diseases are diagnosed by using a list of diagnostic criteria which include both positive and negative criteria. These diagnostic criteria will aim at providing some degree of diagnostic certainty by defining "definite disease" (high specificity) or "probable disease" (high sensitivity). This will help clinicians in treating patients since high-risk treatment modalities should be offered only if the patient has a definite disease; whereas, low-risk treatment can be offered to patients even with probable disease.
The CCBS has set up four disease-specific subcommittees:

- Meniere's disease
- Benign paroxysmal positional vertigo
- Vestibular migraine
- Behavioral neuro-otologic conditions

International Classification of Vestibular Disorders Layer III-B: Mechanisms

Layer III-B contains the pathoanatomic, pathophysiologic, and etiologic mechanisms underlying vestibular disorders. This layer has been created in the hope that ultimately all symptoms and signs may be linked directly with etiological understanding. Major mechanisms include:

- Genetic
- Traumatic
- Inflammatory
- Vascular
- Others

CONCLUSION

Although there are enormous recent innovations in vestibular disorders, the vestibular society may stand behind other neuroscience subspecialties for the simple reason that it lacks the definitive criteria and classification of vestibular disorders. The vestibular society is looking forward to working with other societies to take vestibular research to the next level through consensus criteria for classification and diagnosis.

REFERENCES

1. Bisdorff A, von Brevern M, Lempert T, Newman-Toker DE. Classification of vestibular symptoms: Towards an international classification of vestibular disorders. J Vestib Res. 2009;19(1-2):1-13.
2. Bárány Society. (2015). The International Society for Neuro-Otology. [online] Available from www.baranysociety.nl [Last accessed April, 2025].
3. Bisdorff AR, Staab JP, Newman-Toker DE. Overview of the International Classification of Vestibular Disorders. Neurol Clin. 2015;33(3):541-50.

7
CHAPTER

Peripheral Vertigo: Episodic

Ajit Verma

ABSTRACT

Episodic dizziness is a diagnostically challenging clinical problem, characterized by a wide range of potential causes, overlapping features, and the frequent absence of definitive diagnostic tests or abnormal findings on examination between episodes. The cornerstone of evaluation remains a meticulous clinical history, as symptom quality is often unreliable and physical signs may be absent outside of acute episodes. Vestibular migraine is the most common cause of spontaneous episodic dizziness and is frequently underdiagnosed due to its overlap with conditions like Ménière's disease, panic disorder, and transient ischemic attacks. Accurate diagnosis is critical, as many of these conditions are treatable. This chapter discusses the clinical features, diagnostic considerations, and management strategies for the most common causes of episodic dizziness, emphasizing the value of longitudinal follow-up and multidisciplinary assessment in ambiguous cases.

INTRODUCTION

Episodic dizziness is a frequent clinical presentation that poses significant diagnostic challenges due to its diverse etiologies, overlapping symptoms, and often normal interictal examination findings. Unlike acute continuous vertigo, episodic forms occur in discrete attacks, often without objective findings between episodes. The differential diagnosis spans peripheral vestibular disorders, central nervous system pathologies, cardiovascular conditions, and psychiatric syndromes. This chapter provides a structured overview of common causes of episodic peripheral vertigo, highlighting key clinical features, diagnostic strategies, and treatment approaches. Emphasis is placed on distinguishing characteristics of each condition, red flags for central causes, and the importance of longitudinal follow-up. Understanding the nuanced presentation of episodic vertigo can significantly improve patient outcomes and reduce the burden of unnecessary investigations and delayed treatment.

CLINICAL APPROACH

Episodic dizziness is a challenging problem as there are many causes, overlapping clinical features, and no diagnostic tests. Moreover, symptom quality has been

BOX 1 Episodic spontaneous dizziness.

- Vestibular migraine
- Ménière's disease
- Vertebrobasilar transient ischemic attack
- Vestibular paroxysmia
- Benign recurrent vertigo
- Panic disorder
- Delayed OH
- Cardiogenic dizziness
- Hypoglycemia

found to be unreliable, and clinical examination between the episodes may be normal. History is the key to diagnosis and differential diagnosis. Therefore, history remains the most important aspect of evaluation. **Box 1** shows the most common causes of episodic dizziness.

VESTIBULAR MIGRAINE

Vestibular migraine (VM) is the most common cause of episodic spontaneous dizziness.[1] Though most common and treatable it is most underdiagnosed. The challenges in the diagnosis of VM are, overlapping clinical features [Ménière's disease (MD)], migraine anxiety-related disorders (MARD), isolated and incomplete forms of presentation (benign recurrent vertigo), and sometimes antimigraine drugs producing dizziness. Therefore, VM remains an underdiagnosed entity. VM is seen in the third and fourth decades of life. Migraine headaches typically precede the onset of vertigo by more than a decade. The pathophysiology of VM is incompletely understood. The clinical features of VM can be divided into two categories ictal and interictal. Patients maybe describing vertigo as a false sensation of self-motion or spinning of the surroundings. Though the symptoms are spontaneous they may be aggravated by head motion, visual stimuli, busy patterns, or changing head positions lying down or rolling over. The relationship with headaches is very variable. 50–90% of patients may have associated headaches at least in some of the vestibular episodes. Interestingly other migraine symptoms appear to be more common than headache during vertigo attacks, such as phonophobia and photophobia. Auditory symptoms such as tinnitus and hearing loss can also occur in some patients and can lead to misdiagnosis of MD. Unilateral persistent hearing loss on audiometry is characteristic of MD. Since nausea and vomiting is a symptom of most vestibular disorders it is not considered specific to VM. Duration of VM is highly variable from minutes to hours to days and similarly the frequency of VM few attacks per year two to three per month. Many patients (90%) of VM have a history of motion sickness. There may also be a history of periodic syndromes of childhood, including abdominal pain, cyclic vomiting, BPPV, and benign paroxysmal torticollis, which are considered migraine variants. 50% patients of VM have persistent dizziness labeled as chronic VM, which is more likely a coexisting persistent postural perceptual dizziness (PPPD). In addition to PPPD patients of VM have significant psychological comorbidities of anxiety, depression, and panic. Neuro-otological examination may show spontaneous, gaze-evoked, positional, or other triggered (head shaking or vibration induced) nystagmus. Positional nystagmus is most often persistent, asymptomatic, and central appearing.

Red flags: When patients present for the first time acutely with vestibular symptoms posterior circulation stroke is the most important differential to consider. Presence of direction changing purely torsional or vertical nystagmus. Skew deviation and normal head impulse test and other associated neurological deficits including acute unilateral deafness, dysarthria, limb weakness or incoordination, and severe gait ataxia with inability to walk are highly suggestive of posterior circulation stroke.

Two other differential diagnoses are benign paroxysmal positional vertigo (BPPV) and MD. BPPV is a common cause of recurrent vertigo but should be readily distinguishable from VM given the short duration of vertigo with BPPV (usually 10–30 seconds) provoked by particular head movements. The Dix-Hallpike maneuver is positive in 85% of cases in which the posterior semicircular canal is affected. While the Dix–Hallpike maneuver also provokes nystagmus in VM patients, characteristics of nystagmus are different. In BPPV there is a latency period of a few seconds to onset of nystagmus, which is usually fast velocity, torsional, and fatigues after approximately 30 seconds. In contrast, nystagmus in VM has no latency period, is generally of low velocity, horizontal (although a fifth may be vertical), and sustained.

Suspect VM in younger patients if there is prominent nausea or vomiting, and in those not responding to repositioning maneuvers. The treatment of VM is on the lines of migraine.

MÉNIÈRE'S DISEASE

Ménière's disease affects 1% of the population. The main symptoms of MD are attacks of rotatory vertigo lasting 20 minutes to a few hours accompanied by fluctuating sensorineural hearing loss, tinnitus, and aural fullness. During attacks patients may have nausea, vomiting, tachycardia, and headache, and in chronic stage postural and gait imbalance, BPPV, vestibular drops attacks, and bilateral vestibulopathy. In contrast to idiopathic BPPV, MD-related BPPV more often arises from the horizontal semicircular canal and may require multiple repositioning maneuvers. Vestibular drop attacks lead to a sudden fall on the ground without loss of consciousness, but vestibular drop attacks sometimes trigger loss of consciousness which is vestibular syncope. Depression anxiety is seen in 50% of patients and therefore physicians should screen for these two disorders. Fatigue is also a commonly associated symptom. In the diagnosis of MD audiometry plays an important role. In the early stages it is low frequency hearing loss producing a rising curve is typical. Monosymptomatic forms manifest with either hearing loss or episodes of vertigo and may be difficult to diagnose in the initial stages. Vertigo attacks resembling MD may occur with VM, central nervous system (CNS) inflammatory disorders, transient ischemic attacks (TIAs), and some inner-ear diseases. Conservative management of MD includes lifestyle modification, including reduced salt intake and medication such as diuretics and betahistine. If conservative measures are ineffective, surgical options include intratympanic injections of corticosteroid and gentamicin, endolymphatic sac decompression, and labyrinthectomy.[2,3]

VERTEBROBASILAR TRANSIENT ISCHEMIC ATTACK

Contrary to proper belief isolated vertigo (without diplopia, dysphagia, dysarthria, dysesthesia, and limb weakness) can be a manifestation of vertebrobasilar insufficiency. 50% patients of with posterior circulation stroke have preceding isolated vertigo.[4] Though uncommon it is an important and dangerous condition not to miss. In older people with recent onset of symptoms can be a manifestation of vertebrobasilar TIA. Since the anterior inferior cerebellar artery (AICA) supplies the cochlea and vestibular labyrinth sudden and fluctuating hearing loss may also be due to vascular insufficiency rather than MD. Sudden hearing loss along with vertigo is a risk for subsequent stroke. There is increasing evidence that new hearing loss with acute vestibular syndrome can be a stroke. Therefore, the possibility of vertebrobasilar ischemia should be considered in older patients with risk factors for stroke, especially of recent onset (<3 months), lasting for minutes to one or two hours with or without auditory symptoms. New headaches, neck pain, or recent neck trauma with vertigo may be due to vertebral artery dissection. If the patient comes at a time when he is symptomatic HINTS (Head-Impulse, Nystagmus, Test-of-Skew) plus an examination may be helpful. If not conclusive then symptoms and risk factors ($ABCD^2$) should be evaluated including an angiography to detect vertebrobasilar stenosis.

VESTIBULAR PAROXYSMIA

In this condition, there are brief attacks of vertigo (from one to a few seconds) multiple times per day (one per month to 10–20/day) with or without tinnitus. Usually, attacks are spontaneous but at times triggered by head turned, loud noise, or hyperventilation. As in trigeminal neuralgia, these episodes are due to emphatic transmission between adjacent axons. High-resolution magnetic resonance imaging (MRI)-CISS (Constructive Interference in Steady State)/ FIESTA (Fast Imaging Employing Steady-state Acquisition). Sequence through the brainstem should be performed to demonstrate neurovascular compression and other conditions such as CP angle tumor, arachnoid cyst, demyelinating lesion, or any other structure cause for the episodes. Differential diagnoses of short attacks are BPPV, Otolithic crisis of Tumarkin (MD), paroxysmal brainstem attacks [multiple sclerosis and cerebrovascular accidents (CVA)], and superior canal dehiscence syndrome. For longer-lasting attacks (>5) VM, MD, vertebrobasilar TIAs, and panic attacks should be considered. This disease is highly responsive to carbamazepine, oxcarbazepine, and lacosamide.[5,6]

BENIGN RECURRENT VERTIGO

This condition is characterized by episodes of spontaneous vertigo without migrainous, neurologic, or otologic features that do not go on to cause any persistent vestibular or hearing loss. The majority of these patients fit into the diagnostic criteria of probable VM. Patients have a family history of migraines and 50% develop migraines on follow-up. Some patients of benign recurrent vertigo are found to have recurrent spontaneous vertigo with interictal head-shaking nystagmus.

PANIC ATTACKS

Psychogenic dizziness can be acute as in panic attacks and it can be chronic as in chronic subjective dizziness. Patients with recurrent vestibular dysfunction can present with chronic psychogenic dizziness. A pt may have associated vestibular dysfunction like vestibular neuritis, may have only an abnormal vestibular test, and at times an acute attack of BPPV or VM and trigger a panic attack.

Panic attacks commonly cause dizziness and are only second to cardiopulmonary symptoms which are the most common presentation. Panic attacks are identified on the basis of a characteristic combination of multiple symptoms **Box 2**. Panic attacks may be part of panic disorder, generalized anxiety disorder, or phobias. Panic disorder and anxiety can present with episodic dizziness without vestibular dysfunction. The key feature to diagnose panic disorder is a careful history. Evaluation of suspected panic attacks may need to rule out hypoglycemia, drug intoxication, drug withdrawal, hyperthyroidism, pheochromocytoma, angina, arrhythmias, and temporal lobe epilepsy. Panic disorder is typically managed with cognitive behavior therapy and selective serotonin reuptake inhibitors (SSRIs).

BOX 2 Symptoms.

- Palpitations or accelerated heart rate
- Sweating
- Trembling or shaking
- Sensations of shortness of breath or smothering
- Feeling of choking
- Chest pain or discomfort
- Nausea or abdominal distress
- Feeling dizzy
- Unsteady
- Light-headed or faint
- Derealization (feelings of unreality) or depersonalization (being detached from oneself)
- Fear of losing control or going insane
- Sense of impending death
- Paresthesias
- Chills or hot flushes

A challenging problem of panic disorder-related dizziness is to pick up associated migraine vertigo or BPPV which is a treatable vestibular type of vertigo and can be distinguished from panic attack-related dizziness by the presence of nausea vomiting, history of actual fall, eyewitnesses noticing imbalance, or unsteady gait. Similarly, a patient may have symptoms of presyncope triggered by strong emotions and may be misdiagnosed as a panic attack.

ORTHOSTATIC HYPOTENSION

Orthostatic hypotension (OH) is a common cause of dizziness in 5–30% in the elderly population. It can present with a variety of symptoms such as vertigo, dizziness, light-headedness tiredness, fading vision, posterior head or neck discomfort, tachycardia, and palpitation relieved by sitting or lying down. There may be subtle symptoms such as tiredness, and difficulty in thinking and concentrating. OH is a drop in blood pressure (>20 mm Hg systolic and/or >10 mm Hg diastolic) that occurs within 3 minutes of standing. Orthostatic hypotension is of three types; early (within 15 seconds of standing), classical (within 3 minutes of standing), and delayed (usually, after 3 minutes). In delayed OH the relationship between the trigger (upright posture) and dizziness is not clear to the patient and the patient usually complains of spontaneous dizziness. A number of other conditions that mimic OH are; postural tachycardia syndrome (Potts), PPPD, orthostatic tremor/myoclonus, and gait disturbances. The management of OH is nonpharmacological and pharmacological.[7,8]

CARDIOGENIC VERTIGO

Rotational vertigo is considered a typical symptom of vestibular dysfunction but interestingly it could be a manifestation of cardiac disease with serious consequences. The clinical features of cardiogenic vertigo other than vertigo are presyncope, dizziness, syncope lightheadedness, chest discomfort, and breathlessness. These patients are usually above 60 years old with cardiovascular risks, such as hypertension diabetes, and smoking. The dizziness or vertigo lasts seconds to minutes. The most common cause is bradycardia including sick sinus syndrome, tachycardia-bradycardia syndrome, and complete atrioventricular block, others are ischemic cardiomyopathy, atrial fibrillation angina, and valvular heart disease.[9,10]

Summary

Spontaneous dizziness is a common problem. The most common cause is VM. Persistent hearing loss on audiometry is a clue to MD. Auditory symptoms occur not only in MD but also in migraine and AICA TIAs and strokes. Multiple attacks per day (20–30) short duration is highly suggestive of vestibular paroxysmia an uncommon but potentially treatable cause. Many patients of spontaneous dizziness/vertigo may not fit into a well-defined diagnostic category on the first consultation. Young patients diagnosed with benign recurrent vertigo may later turn out to be VM. Following the patient over a few months is very rewarding (always following your patient is a golden rule with very helpful results). Isolated vertigo due to vertebrobasilar insufficiency, though uncommon but important and should be considered in patients with stroke risk factors, even when other brainstem symptoms are not there. Variety and a long list of somatic symptoms (though overbearing in a busy outdoors) is a helpful diagnostic clue to anxiety and panic disorder.

CONCLUSION

Episodic dizziness is a prevalent yet complex clinical complaint requiring careful evaluation and longitudinal observation. Vestibular migraine emerges as the leading cause, often underrecognized due to its variable symptomatology and overlap with other vestibular and systemic disorders. Persistent hearing loss favors a diagnosis of Ménière's disease, while brief, repetitive attacks may point toward vestibular paroxysmia. Cardiovascular and psychiatric causes must also be considered, particularly in older patients or those with risk factors. Therefore, structured follow-up and patient education are vital. Treatment should be individualized, addressing not only vestibular dysfunction but also comorbid conditions such as anxiety and depression. Ultimately, the nuanced evaluation of episodic dizziness demands a balance of clinical vigilance, diagnostic acumen, and empathic longitudinal care.

REFERENCES

1. Li V, McArdle H, Trip SA. Vestibular migraine. BMJ. 2019;366:l4213.
2. Hamid A. A Mohamed. Meniere's disease Pract Neurol. 2009;9(3):157-62.
3. Kutlubaev MA, Pyykko I, Hardy TA, Gürkov R. Meniere's disease Pract. Neurol. 2020;1-6.
4. Lee H, Sohn SI, Jung DK, Cho YW, Lim JG, Yi SD, et al. Sudden deafness and anterior inferior cerebellar artery infarction. Stroke. 2002;33(12):2807-12.
5. Strupp M, Lopez-Escamez JA, Kim JS, Straumann D, Jen JC, Carey J, et al. Vestibular paroxysmia: Diagnostic criteria. J Vestib Res. 2016;26(5-6): 409-15.
6. Hufner K, Barresi D, Glaser M, Linn J, Adrion C, Mansmann U, et al. Vestibular paroxysmia: diagnostic features and medical treatment. Neurology. 2008;71(13):1006-14.
7. Gilani A, Juraschek SP, Belanger MJ, Vowles JE, Wannamethee SG. Postural hypotension. BMJ. 2021;373:n922.
8. Mader SL. Identification and management of orthostatic hypotension in older and medically complex patients. Expert Rev Cardiovasc Ther. 2012;10(3):387-95.
9. Kim AH, Ahn J, Park HS, Lee SM, Choi SY, Oh EH, et al. Cardiogenic vertigo: characteristics and proposed diagnostic criteria. J Neurol. 2021;268(3):1070-5.
10. Newman-Toker DE, Camargo CA Jr. 'Cardiogenic vertigo'—true vertigo as the presenting manifestation of primary cardiac disease. Nat Clin Pract Neurol. 2006;2(3):167-72.

8 CHAPTER Peripheral Vertigo (Episodic): Benign Paroxysmal Positional Vertigo

Rithvik Ramesh, Ajay Kumar Vats, Venkata Sai Suhas Yadlapati

ABSTRACT

Benign paroxysmal positional vertigo (BPPV) is the most common peripheral vestibular disorder characterized by brief episodes of vertigo provoked by specific changes in head position. It arises from mechanical disruption within the semicircular canals due to displaced otoconia from the utricle, leading to abnormal stimulation of the vestibular system. Understanding the anatomical and physiological basis of the semicircular canals and their role in the vestibulo-ocular reflex is essential for accurate diagnosis. This chapter explores the canal-specific physics of endolymph flow and the differential effects of otolithic debris in various BPPV subtypes—posterior, horizontal, and anterior canal involvement.

INTRODUCTION

Benign paroxysmal positional vertigo (BPPV) is a common cause of dizziness and brief episodes of vertigo, often triggered by changes in head position. It arises from disturbances in the inner ear, specifically when small calcium particles interfere with the physiological endolymphatic flow within the semicircular canals. The initial severity can be debilitation causing a lot of panic in the patients.[1] Understanding the anatomy and function of these canals, along with the physics behind the fluid movement and its effects, is essential for diagnosing and managing BPPV. Through specific maneuvers, clinicians can observe telltale signs of the disorder, guiding effective treatment.

ANATOMY AND SOME EAR PHYSICS

To understand BPPV, and its associated eye movements and maneuvers, understanding the anatomy of the inner ear, with some physics is mandatory. The organs of balance and hearing are essentially housed within a set of interlocked canals and cavities within the bony labyrinth, inside which is the membranous labyrinth. This comprises the bony cochlea, with the *cochlear duct* inside, the vestibule with the *utricle and saccule inside,* and the three semicircular canals, with the *semicircular ducts* inside.[2] As discussed in Chapter 1, there are three canals oriented to detect angular acceleration in different planes. Common to these canals is that they are filled with endolymph and have a dilated sac at one end called the ampulla which contains the crista ampullaris, consisting of the cupula and the stereocilia (hair cells). The cupula is a gelatinous component that extends from the crista to the roof of the ampulla. Based on the direction of flow of endolymph, the cupula bends which determines the net stimulation or inhibition of hair cells of that canal, which are conducted to the vestibular nerve.

Physiologically each canal works to stabilize the vision in response to angular head movements in a particular direction. This stabilization of vision occurs as each canal has distinct oculomotor connections. Which direction of head movement would be stimulatory is dependent on the individual canal, as each canal is maximally sensitive for rotations around an axis perpendicular to the plane of that canal and when in the direction of that canal.[3] Additionally, each canal works in tandem with its partner canal on the opposite side of the head. This is summarized in **Table 1**.

When the head is moved in a particular direction, say for instance toward the right before crossing a road, many factors come into play internally. Both horizontal semicircular canals (HSCC) are affected but in opposite ways due to their mirrored orientation.

TABLE 1: Canal position, and its connections.

Canal	Position	Stimulatory movement	Tandem canal	Connections	Eye movement
Posterior SCC	Vertical, posterior	Head tilting backward and toward the same side	Anterior SCC (contralateral)	*Posterior SCC* → *Vestibular nerve (inferior division)* → *Vestibular nuclei* → *Contralateral oculomotor nucleus* (via MLF) → *Superior oblique* and *inferior rectus* muscles	Torsional (top of the eye rotates toward the nose) and vertical (downward) movement
Anterior SCC	Vertical, anterior	Head tilting forward and toward the same side	Posterior SCC (contralateral)	*Anterior SCC* → *Vestibular nerve* (superior division) → *Vestibular nuclei* → *Contralateral oculomotor nucleus* (via MLF) → *Superior rectus and inferior oblique* muscles	Torsional (top of the eye rotates away from the nose) and vertical (upward) movement
Horizontal SCC	Horizontal, lateral	Head turning to the same side (left or right)	Horizontal SCC (contralateral)	*Horizontal SCC* → *Vestibular nerve* (superior division) → *Vestibular nuclei* → *Contralateral abducens nucleus* (via MLF) → *Lateral rectus* muscle (ipsilateral) and *medial rectus* muscle (contralateral via oculomotor nerve)	Horizontal movement (side-to-side)

Movement of the Endolymph and its Effect on the Cupula

When the head is turned to the right, the bony part of the semicircular canal moves with your head, but the endolymph inside the canal lags behind due to *inertia*. Inertia is a fundamental concept in Newtonian physics that refers to the tendency of an object to resist changes in its state of motion. This means that an object at rest will stay at rest, and an object in motion will continue moving at a constant velocity (in a straight line) unless acted upon by an external force. It is determined by the mass of the substance, i.e., the more the mass more inertia it exerts.[4] This concept will be revisited later.

This lag of endolymph causes the endolymph in both horizontal canals to move in the opposite direction of your head movement relative to the canals or more accurately remain stationary relative to the motion of the bony canals. So specifically, during the right head turn movement, the endolymph in the right horizontal canal appears to move toward the ampulla called ampullopetal flow (when actually the bony canal moves toward the lagging endolymph), while in the left horizontal canal, it appears to move away from the ampulla, i.e., ampullofugal flow (when actually the bony canal moves away from the lagging endolymph).[5]

The flow of endolymph causes the cupula to bend. Based on the above example, in the right horizontal canal there is ampullopetal flow of the endolymph causing the cupula to bend toward the utricle. In the left horizontal canal, there is ampullofugal flow causing the cupula to bend away from the utricle. This cupula and endolymph movement has stimulatory or inhibitory effects depending on the individual semicircular canal and has been established by Ewald's laws, specifically 2 and 3, based on the direction of bending of the cupula and the kinocilia.[6]

- *Ewald''s second law*: In the horizontal canal, ampullopetal flow (toward the ampulla) causes a stronger response than ampullofugal flow.
- *Ewald's third law*: In the anterior and posterior canals, ampullofugal flow (away from the ampulla) causes a stronger response than ampullopetal flow.

Now based on this, the ampullopetal flow in the right HSCC is stimulatory and the ampullofugal flow in the left HSCC ends up being inhibitory. This right HSCC-induced stimulation causes activation of the left lateral rectus and the right medial rectus muscles, causing the eyes to move left, which is the opposite direction to the movement of the head in this example, thereby maintaining visual fixation. This entire reflex is the vestibulo-ocular reflex (VOR), and it is when this process through the semicircular canals is affected, it leads to BPPV.

PATHOGENESIS AND ETIOLOGY

The pathophysiology in BPPV is attributed to otoconia, which are calcium carbonate crystals that are normally found attached to the hair cells of the utricle. These, when dislodged enter the semicircular canals (canalolithiasis) or get attached to the cupula (cupulolithiasis). When they reach a sufficient amount to alter the mass of the endolymph or cupula, they alter the inertia or stiffness of the respective structure. In canalolithiasis the debris can fall toward or away from the ampulla, creating ampullopetal or ampullofugal deflection of the cupula by a pump or suction mechanism, or by the hydrodynamic drag. When the otoconia adheres to the cupula it makes it stiffer, and more sensitive to the gravitational forces.[7] The detached otoconia, has a higher predilection for the posterior canals, because of its anatomic orientation, such that when the patient lies flat, the nonampullary orifice of the posterior semicircular canal (PSCC) is lower than the utricle. As to why the otoconia detach in the first place, many causes have been explored including spontaneous detachment and entry. **Table 2** lists the possible secondary causes of BPPV.[8]

Based on the SCC involved and the limb, and the type of BPPC can be categorized as shown in **Figure 1**.

TABLE 2: Causes of BPPV.

Post-traumatic: • Minor head trauma • Craniofacial trauma	*Otological disorders*: • Ménière's disease • Acute vestibular syndrome
Postprocedural: • Dental and maxillofacial • Middle ear surgeries • Cochlear implant	*Vitamin D deficiency*: • *Vascular:* ○ Migraine ○ Giant cell arteritis
• Migraine • Age • Hypertension • Diabetes mellitus	

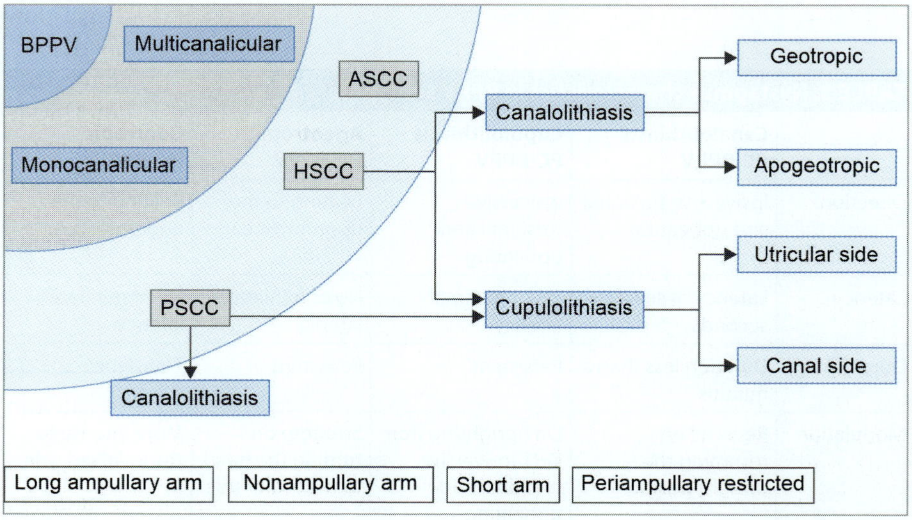

FIG. 1: Classification of BPPV.

(ASCC: anterior semicircular canal; BPPV: benign paroxysmal positional vertigo; HSCC: horizontal semicircular canal; PSCC: posterior semicircular canal)

DIAGNOSIS

Clinically symptoms that are suggestive of BPPV, are when the dizziness is episodic, positional, and transient usually seconds. Other differentials including orthostatic hypotension, perilymphatic fistula, superior canal dehiscence, central positional nystagmus, bow hunter syndrome, and even vestibular migraine have to be considered. More specifically, vertigo that occurs on waking up, meaning that it is associated with more vertical head movements could denote posterior canal BPPV or rarely anterior canal BPPV. Vertigo which awakes from sleep, meaning possibly triggered by side-to-side head movement could indicate horizontal canal BPPV, but these findings have to be interpreted cautiously after positional tests. Additionally, vertigo associated with a lot of autonomic features could indicate horizontal canal BPPV as well.[9,10] At the onset, vertigo episodes tend to be severe but gradually lessen in intensity over time. In the early stages, nausea or vomiting often accompanies the vertigo, and patients may overestimate the duration of each episode. The early active phase of BPPV can last for days to even months. It usually resolves on its own with frequent recurrences. In chronic cases where the active phase continues, the condition becomes intractable with patients reporting a sensation of floating or unsteadiness in posture. But beyond these symptomatic reasoning, BPPV is assessed and diagnosed by performing positional tests, specific to each canal and is diagnosed based on the generated oculomotor responses during positional tests **(Table 3)** and will be elaborated underneath.

Posterior Canal

Posterior semicircular canal dysfunction is assessed by the Dix–Hallpike maneuver or the side-lying test for BPPV (Semont diagnostic maneuver).

TABLE 3: Nystagmus characteristics in BPPV subtypes.

	Canalolithiasis PC-BPPV	Cupulolithiasis PC-BPPV	Ageotropic HC-BPPV	Geotropic HC-BPPV
Direction	Ipsiversive torsional and upbeating	Ipsiversive torsional and upbeating	Beating to the uppermost ear	Beating to the undermost ear
Latency	Latency of several seconds	No or minimal latency	No or minimal latency	No or minimal latency
Duration	Duration less than a minute	Persistent	Persistent	Transient
Modulation	Reversal on resuming the upright position	On uprighting from DHT ipsiversive torsional and upbeating	Stronger on turning the head to the intact side	More intense to the involved side
Fatigability	Fatigability++	Less fatigable	Less fatigable	Fatigable

(BPPV: benign paroxysmal positional vertigo; DHT: Dix–Hallpike test)

Diagnostic Steps in the Dix–Hallpike Maneuver

- *Patient starts in a seated position*:
  - *Why*: This position is the baseline, allowing the examiner to observe the patient's eyes and reactions before moving into the testing phase. It also provides a stable position to transition from when testing each side.
- *The head is rotated 45° toward the examiner*:
  - *Why*: *By rotating the head, the PSCC of the affected ear is aligned parallel to the sagittal plane, and the ampullary end is positioned rostrally. This positioning makes the* canal most susceptible to the gravitational pull when the head is moved downward.
- *Patient is rapidly laid back into a supine position with the head hyperextended to 20º*:
  - *Why*: *This rapid movement encourages the otoconia (if present) to shift within the* PSCC. The head is placed lower than the rest of the body, with the neck hyperextended to enhance this displacement. The otoconia are now displaced to the most dependent position from their initial position. The ampulla is also taken to a higher position.
    - In *long ampullary arm PSCC canalolithiasis,* which is the most common type, this maneuver now displaces the particles in an ampullofugal direction, which causes a plunger effect and increased cumulative inertia of the endolymph by itself, causing the cupula to deflect away from the utricle (cupular stimulation, refer to Ewald's third law), leading to ipsitorsional upbeating nystagmus. (Patients view). This is paroxysmal and fatigable.
- In *cupulolithiasis,* the nystagmus is persistent, reflecting the adherence of otolithic debris. Moreover, there is a stronger response when the patient lies flat, as the cupula becomes maximally stimulated by gravity. The *Half-Hallpike test (HHT)* is performed similarly to the Dix–Hallpike test (DHT), with a key modification in the degree of movement. The patient's head initially rotated 45° from the upright long-sitting position, is lowered to 60° in the supine position rather than the full 120° used in the DHT. A pillow approximately 4" thick is placed at the head end of the examination table. This supports the head in a position of approximately 30° of anteflexion, achieving the necessary positioning for the HHT. In cases where the HHT elicits an upbeating ipsitorsional nystagmus (UBITN) lasting longer than one minute, *a positive inversion test* is employed. This test involves positioning the patient in a contralateral recumbent position with the nose down. A transition from UBITN to downbeating contratorsional nystagmus (DBCTN) suggests the presence of cupulolithiasis, particularly of the adherent type.
- In *nonampullary arm PSC canalolithiasis,* also called the apogeotropic PSC BPPV otoconia are free-floating in the nonampullary arm near the common crus. So, when the head is lowered during DHM, the debris moves to the dependent position, thereby producing a hydrostatic ampullopetal flow, causing cupula deflection toward the ampulla causing inhibition. This causes a contratorsional and downbeating nystagmus. A downbeating torsional nystagmus can also suggest ASC-BPPV.

- *Holding the position for 20–30 seconds*:
  Why: This step is necessary because the nystagmus and vertigo may not appear immediately. The delay (latency period) allows time for the otoconia to move within the canal and trigger the positional nystagmus and vertigo.
- *Returning to the seated position*:
  Why: The patient is then returned to the seated position with the head still rotated, causing the reverse movement of the otoconia. During this reversal, the direction of the nystagmus and vertigo also reverses, but the intensity is typically less than in the initial phase. When returning to the sitting position, the otoconia now moves in the ampullopetal direction (toward the utricle), causing an inhibitory response. The reversal of nystagmus (now downbeating with torsion) reflects this inhibitory effect. Upbeating ipsitorsional nystagmus on sitting up from DHT indicates PSC-BPPV in the short arm.
- *Repeat on the other side*:
  Variations: An alternative to the Dix–Hallpike test is the Semont diagnostic maneuver, also known as the "side-lying" test. This maneuver mirrors the initial step of the Semont therapeutic procedure. It is especially beneficial when the examiner is already aware of the affected side and wishes to confirm whether the positional nystagmus has resolved following treatment.

Horizontal Canal

The horizontal canal (lateral canal) is the second most commonly affected canal in BPPV. Unlike posterior canal BPPV, where torsional and vertical nystagmus are common, horizontal canal BPPV is characterized by direction-changing horizontal nystagmus. The McClure–Pagnini test (also known as the supine roll test or head yaw test) is the primary diagnostic maneuver for horizontal canal BPPV.

Diagnostic Steps for Horizontal Canal BPPV Supine Head Roll (LC-BPPV)

- *Look for spontaneous nystagmus with the patient seated*:
  Why: In some cases, horizontal canal BPPV can present with pseudo-spontaneous nystagmus due to otoconia close to or attached to the cupula, which can be modulated by head shaking. Observing this in the seated position gives an initial clue to the involvement of the horizontal canal. If spontaneous nystagmus is present then changes in the nystagmus direction, position or intensity can be looked for by bending the head about 30 and 60° forward and then 60° backward.
- *The patient is then placed in the supine position with the head straight and slightly elevated by 30° (to align the horizontal canals in the vertical plane). The patient's head is rolled 90° to one side, and then 180° to the other side.*
  Why: Rolling the head causes the otoconia to move within the canal, creating an endolymphatic flow that displaces the cupula either toward (ampullopetal) or away (ampullofugal) from the utricle. This flow stimulates the vestibular system, causing horizontal nystagmus.
- In geotropic nystagmus (the most common form), otoconia are free-floating in the horizontal canal and move toward the lowest part of the canal during

head rotation, causing ampullopetal flow due to hydrodynamic drag. This stimulates the cupula and causes intense nystagmus toward the ground. When the head is rotated to the other side, the debris moves away from the ampulla (ampullofugal flow), causing a weaker inhibitory response, and thus, less intense nystagmus in the opposite direction.

  - The side that elicits the more intense nystagmus during lateral head roll is the affected side.

- In apogeotropic nystagmus (less common), the otoconia are either attached to the cupula or close to the ampulla, making it more sensitive to positional changes. When the head is turned, the cupula becomes deflected in the direction of gravity, causing ampullofugal deflection of the ipsilateral cupula, resulting in its inhibition, with excitation of the opposite HC causing apogeotropic nystagmus, where the nystagmus beats away from the ground. The side which during lateral head roll elicits the weaker nystagmus is the affected side.
- *Test for bow and lean signs (bow and lean test)*:
  Why: This test further helps to differentiate between the geotropic and apogeotropic forms of horizontal canal BPPV and assists in identifying the affected ear. The patient's head is bent forward (bow) by 30° and then leaned back (lean) by 60°.
- In geotropic LC-BPPV, bow nystagmus is directed toward the affected side, and lean nystagmus is directed away from the affected side.
- In apogeotropic LC-BPPV, the bow and lean test produces the opposite effects, with nystagmus lean nystagmus directed toward the affected ear and bow nystagmus directed away from the affected ear.

Anterior Canal

Anterior canal BPPV (AC-BPPV) is much rarer than posterior or horizontal canal BPPV, yet it can still be detected through specific diagnostic maneuvers. Due to the positioning of the anterior canal (AC) relative to the posterior canal (PC) of the opposite side, testing the posterior canal also indirectly stimulates the contralateral anterior canal. The primary maneuvers used to diagnose AC-BPPV include the Dix-Hallpike maneuver and the head-hanging test.

Diagnostic Steps for Anterior Canal Benign Paroxysmal Positional Vertigo

- *Dix-Hallpike maneuver (left side for right AC)*:
  Why: When testing for anterior canal BPPV, the contralateral Dix-Hallpike maneuver (e.g., left-sided Dix-Hallpike for right anterior canal) is used, as the anterior canal is co-planar with the opposite side's posterior canal.
  If the right anterior canal is affected, performing the left-sided Dix-Hallpike maneuver provokes ampullofugal flow in the left anterior canal, causing downbeating nystagmus with a torsional component (top pole beating toward the affected ear). The debris causes endolymph to move in the ampullofugal (excitatory) direction, stimulating the anterior canal and its associated vestibulo-ocular reflex pathways.

- *Straight head-hanging test*: The patient is laid in the supine position with the head hanging 30° below horizontal.
    - *Why*: This test is often more sensitive for detecting anterior canal BPPV than the Dix–Hallpike maneuver due to the vertical orientation of the anterior canal. The straight head-hanging position allows gravitational forces to stimulate the anterior canal directly. The otoconia moves toward the ampulla in an ampullopetal direction, stimulating the anterior canal and causing downbeating nystagmus with a torsional component.

In anterior canal BPPV, the characteristic nystagmus is typically downbeating with a possible torsional component (though this is often very little and difficult to detect). The intensity of the nystagmus may be lower compared to posterior canal BPPV, and it may not reverse when returning the patient to the sitting position.

Many patients can present with multicanalicular BPPV, which can be unilateral and bilateral requiring careful assessment of positional test.

Treatment of BPPV is detailed in Chapters 13 and 14.

CONCLUSION

A comprehensive understanding of BPPV begins with understanding the anatomy and functional physiology of the semicircular canals. The condition exemplifies how a mechanical disruption, such as dislodged otoconia, can produce distinct clinical signs and positional nystagmus patterns based on canal orientation and endolymph dynamics. Each subtype—posterior, horizontal, or anterior canal BPPV—has characteristic diagnostic features which, when correctly identified through maneuvers like the Dix–Hallpike or supine roll test, allow for precise localization and pathophysiological categorization. While the initial episodes may be debilitating, the condition is largely benign and responds well to repositioning therapies when accurately diagnosed. This chapter underscores the importance of a structured, canal-oriented diagnostic approach, enabling improved diagnostic accuracy and guiding effective therapeutic strategies for patients with positional vertigo.

REFERENCES

1. Kim JS, Zee DS. Clinical practice. Benign paroxysmal positional vertigo. N Engl J Med. 2014;370(12):1138-47.
2. Ekdale EG. Form and function of the mammalian inner ear. J Anat. 2016;228(2):324-37.
3. Cohen B, Tokumasu K, Goto K. Semicircular canal nerve eye and head movements. The Effect of Changes in Initial Eye and Head Position on the Plane of the Induced Movement. Arch Ophthalmol. 1966;76(4):523-31.
4. Freeman DM, Weiss TF. The role of fluid inertia in mechanical stimulation of hair cells. Hear Res. 1988;35(2-3):201-7.
5. Rabbitt RD. Semicircular canal biomechanics in health and disease. J Neurophysiol. 2019;121(3):732-55.
6. In: Ewald JR, University College, London Library Services (Eds). Physiologische Untersuchungen ueber das Endorgan des Nervus Octavus. Wiesbaden: Bergman JF; 1892.
7. Yetiser S. Review of the pathology underlying benign paroxysmal positional vertigo. J Int Med Res. 2020;48(4):300060519892370.

8. Guerra J, Devesa J. Causes and treatment of idiopathic benign paroxysmal positional vertigo based on endocrinological and other metabolic factors. J Otol. 2020;15(4):155-60.
9. Vats AK. The Clinical Spectrum of Patients of Horizontal Semicircular Canal Benign Paroxysmal Positional Vertigo Attending an Otoneurology Center in South Rajasthan, India and Their Response to Appropriate Repositioning Maneuvers at a Short-term Follow-up. Annal Otol Neurotol. 2020;3(02):61-71.
10. Vadlamani S, Dorasala S, Dutt SN. Diagnostic Positional Tests and Therapeutic Maneuvers in the Management of Benign Paroxysmal Positional Vertigo. Indian J Otolaryngol Head Neck Surg. 2022;74(Suppl 1):475-87.

9 CHAPTER Persistent Dizziness

Noel James, Nirumal Khumar

ABSTRACT

This article reviews causes of persistent dizziness. These disorders which were previously included under the term "functional dizziness" have now been reclassified under this category of persisting dizziness. It includes persistent postural perceptual dizziness (PPPD), Mal de debarquement syndrome, dizziness related to concussion, motion sickness and bilateral vestibulopathy. To make a diagnosis of PPPD, its expected to meet Bárány Society criteria. PPPD usually starts as a episodic vertigo, then progresses to peristent dizziness. Mal de debarquement is diagnosed when a patient develops persistent dizziness after prolonged air or ship travel. Persistent dizziness after concussion is classified as structural and nonstructural causes. Motion sickness is a very common problem encountered on a daily basis. The pathogensis implicated is mismatch of sensory inputs. It can be managed with short term vestibular suppressants taken few minutes before travel. Non-pharmacological measures include avoiding mobile phones during travel and changing orientation to facing it to the direction of vehicle movements. Bilateral vestibulopathy is a result of drugs toxins, infectious or autoimmune process. The main mode of treatment of persistent dizziness is vestibular rehabilitation which when done on a long term basis helps with the symptoms and balance.

INTRODUCTION

Persistent dizziness or chronic vestibular syndrome is a syndrome of vertigo and dizziness lasting months to years. The usual symptoms include gait unsteadiness, ataxia, hearing loss, nausea, and oscillopsia.

The causes may include central and peripheral causes. Symptoms may often begin as an episodic vestibular syndrome and evolve to chronic vestibular syndrome.[1]

The causes of persistent dizziness include:

- Persistent postural perceptual dizziness
- Mal de débarquement (MdDS) syndrome
- Persistent dizziness after mild concussion
- Bilateral vestibulopathy
- Motion sickness and visually-induced motions sickness

PERSISTENT POSTURAL PERCEPTUAL DIZZINESS

Persistent postural perceptual dizziness (PPPD) was defined in 2015 prior to which it was referred to as phobic postural vertigo, space motion discomfort (SMD), visual vertigo, and chronic subjective dizziness. International classification of vestibular disorders defined PPPD in 2017 as unsteadiness and nonvertiginous dizziness, which is present for more than 90 days, which is exacerbated by positions such as walking, sitting upright, standing, or complex visual stimuli.[2]

The term phobic postural vertigo has now been dissociated from PPPD as it is considered a primary mood disorder in the spectrum of obsessive-compulsive disorders.[1]

The criteria established by Bárány Society for International Classification are mentioned in **Box 1**. The mechanism and disease course are represented in **Flowchart 1**.

Mechanism and Course

Even though patients with PPPD complain of constant unsteadiness, they rarely fall. Presence of fall is reg flag against the diagnosis of PPPD.

BOX 1 Criteria for persistent postural perceptual dizziness (PPPD).[3]

Persistent postural perceptual dizziness is defined by criteria A–E. All must be fulfilled:

A. One or more symptoms of dizziness, unsteadiness, or nonspinning vertigo are present for 3 months or more:
   1. Symptoms lasting for hours but may wax and wane in severity
   2. Symptoms need not be present throughout the day

B. Persistent symptoms occur without specific provocation but are exacerbated by 3 factors:
   1. Upright posture
   2. Active or passive motion without regard to direction or position
   3. Exposure to moving visual stimuli or complex visual patterns

C. The disorder is precipitated with conditions that cause vertigo, dizziness or unsteadiness, or problems with balance including acute, episodic, or chronic vestibular syndrome:
   1. When the precipitant is acute or episodic condition, symptoms may settle into the pattern of criteria as the precipitant resolves, but may occur intermittently at first, then settle into a persistent course
   2. When precipitant is a chronic syndrome, symptoms may develop slowly at first and worsen gradually

D. Symptoms cause significant functional distress or functional impairment

E. Symptoms are better accounted by another disease or disorder

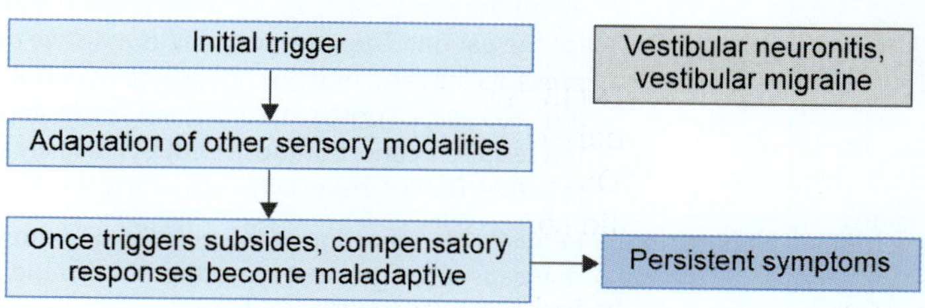

FLOWCHART 1: Pathogenesis of persistent postural perceptual dizziness (PPPD).

Treatment

Three treatment strategies can be used namely (1) vestibular rehabilitation, (2) cognitive behavioral therapy, and (3) serotonergic antidepressant.

Vestibular Rehabilitation

As evidenced by the mechanism, PPPD occurs due to inappropriate sensory weighting to somatosensory or visual cues. Hence, retraining with vestibular rehabilitation improves the symptoms. These rehabilitation measures are usually patient-based. Anxiety, which is a usual comorbidity of PPPD, has to be treated separately and it may even preclude vestibular rehabilitation.[4] The commonly used vestibular rehabilitation measures are outlined in **Table 1**.

Cognitive Behavioral Therapy

The pathological process in PPPD as previously described involves maladaptation to the initial triggering process once the trigger resolves. Hence, avoidance behavior, fearful thoughts, and repeated self-checking behavior form the vicious

TABLE 1: Vestibular rehabilitation strategies.[5]

Rehabilitation for enhancing gaze stability	Adaptation	*Head turns*: While fixing at a stationary object
		Head–trunk turns: The patient looks at his own thumb kept in front with an outstretched arm, while being turned seated on a rotating chair
	Substitution	*Saccade modification*: Corrective saccades act as the main compensatory tactic to replace the defective slow-phase movement
		Enhancement of smooth pursuit movements: • The gains of smooth pursuit movements are higher in patients with vestibulopathy • Smooth pursuit movements take the place of VOR in order to maintain visual fixation
Rehabilitation for enhancing postural stability	Adaptation	*Ankle strategy*: The patient stands with a wide base and sways back and forth and side-to-side with small amplitude movements without allowing motion at the hip or knee
		Hip strategy: The patient stands with a narrow base and does alternate forward bending with ankles dorsiflexed and bends backward with ankle plantar flexed
	Substitution	Use of a cane to provide proprioceptive information about the surface acts as an extension of the finger for the patient. Thus, use of canes as assistive devices prevents falls and must be advocated in people with BVP >65 years. Those with unilateral vestibulopathy do not require a cane, but those with BVP usually require assistive devices, especially in the early stages
Improving vertigo	Habituation	Requires identification of the position and movement that causes the greatest symptoms. Not found to be very helpful in patients with BVP

TABLE 2: Dosing of selective serotonin reuptake inhibitors (SSRI) and selective noradrenergic reuptake inhibitors (SNRI) in persistent postural perceptual dizziness (PPPD).[9]		
Drug class	**Starting dose**	**Therapeutic dose**
Sertraline	25 mg	50–150 mg
Escitalopram	5 mg	10–20 mg/day
Fluoxetine	10 mg	20–60 mg/day
Venlafaxine (SNRI)	37.5 mg	75–225 mg
Duloxetine	20–30 mg	40–60 mg
Mirtazapine	7.5 mg at night	10–30 at night

cycle of PPPD.[6] Cognitive behavioral therapy (CBT) provides benefit in patients with PPPD by helping reduce excessive internal physical alertness. Meta-analysis showed that CBT is of benefit in patients with PPPD when combined with other treatment measures like vestibular rehabilitation and medical therapy.[7]

Medical Therapy

Selective serotonin reuptake inhibitors (SSRIs) and selective noradrenergic reuptake inhibitors (SNRI) are helpful in patients with PPPD.[2]

They help with anxiety component of PPPD but doses are usually one-fourth to half of that used in patients with depression and requires slower titration. This is because starting at higher doses and titrating faster will contribute to existing maladaptation. Clinical effects start to appear only after 2–3 months. Despite these observations, meta-analysis done in 2023 showed that SSRI/SNRI showed no demonstrable effect as compared to placebo.[8]

The dosing of SSRI and SNRI in PPPD is mentioned in **Table 2**.

MAL DE DÉBARQUEMENT SYNDROME

Mal de débarquement syndrome refers to feeling of rocking or swaying that occurs after prolonged exposure to motion.[2] It is usually described in patients who have a recent history of ship travel. The symptoms usually begin after disembarking and may be self-limiting or persistent.

Clinical History

Mal de débarquement syndrome is common in woman usually in their 40s. This usually occurs after a period of passive motion usually after disembarking from an ocean cruise. The common descriptions used by patients include sense of rocking or swaying. There usually is not any sense of spinning, nausea, or vomiting. The symptoms tend to improve when re-exposed to passive motion as in travelling in a car but return when returning to land. The criteria have been mentioned in **Box 2**. **Flowchart 2** gives the pathogenesis of MdDS.

BOX 2 Barany society diagnostic criteria for mal de débarquement syndrome (MdDS).[10]

A. A nonspinning vertigo characterized by oscillatory perception ("rocking", "bobbing", or "swaying") present continuously or for most of the day
B. Onset occurs within 48 hours after the end of exposure to passive motion
C. Symptoms temporarily reduce with exposure to passive motion
D. Symptoms continue for >48 hours:
   - D0: MdDS in evolution—symptoms are ongoing observation period has been less than a month
   - D1: Transient MdDS—symptoms resolve within a month and the observation period was till the time of resolution
   - D2: Persistent MdDS—symptoms last for >1 month

E. Symptoms not better accounted by any other disease or disorder

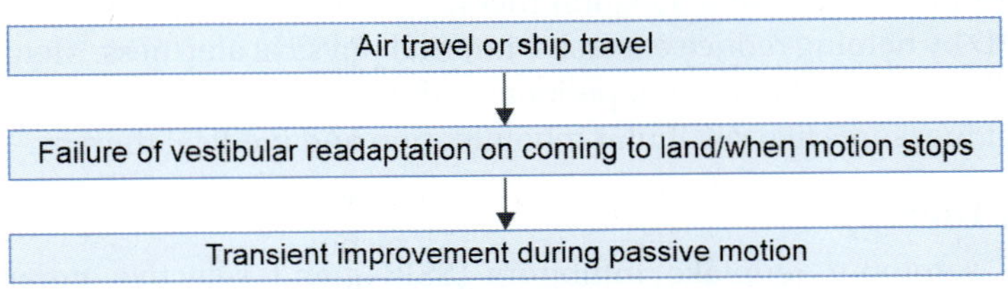

FLOWCHART 2: Pathophysiology of mal de débarquement syndrome.[11]

Laboratory Diagnosis and Differential Diagnosis

Mal de débarquement syndrome is a clinical diagnosis and there is no single lab test which will help with the diagnosis. High index of suspicion is necessary to make a diagnosis.

The common differentials for MdDS are discussed in **Table 3**.

Treatment

The measures that are beneficial for MdDS include lifestyle modifications, transcranial magnetic stimulation, and drugs. But these treatment measures are not effective in all patients with MdDS.

Patients with MdDS frequently feel overwhelmed by open spaces but feel unstable in closed spaces. Low light, noisy environment tends to worsen symptoms, and hence, should be avoided.

Two medications with proven role in MdDS are benzodiazepines and SSRIs. Long-acting benzodiazepines like clonazepam are usually started at 0.25 mg and may be tittered up to 0.5 mg BD.[2]

Intermediate-acting benzodiazepines (lorazepam and diazepam) may be used as preventive therapy before travel. 0.5–1 mg diazepam may be used for this purpose. Flights longer than 6 hours usually require a second dose mid-flight.

The SSRI helps with the symptoms of MdDS and is usually more helpful than noradrenergic agents like tricyclic antidepressants and SNRIs.

Among SNRI, venlafaxine is useful especially in patients who have comorbid migraine.[2]

TABLE 3: Differential diagnosis for mal de débarquement syndrome (MdDS).[11]			
Feature	**MdDS**	**Vestibular migraine**	**PPPD10**
Onset	Abrupt following boat or air travel	Spontaneous, may follow some food triggers	Usually triggered by an inciting event such as BPPV or vestibular migraine
Presence of migraine	Same as normal population	Yes	Same as normal population
Description of vertigo	Rocking, floating, and swaying	Spinning, rocking, and nausea often present	Spinning on exposure to visual stimuli
Examination	Normal	Normal but may have some unsteadiness on Romberg test	Usually, normal
Response to medication	No	Responds to migraine treatment	Responds to SSRI/SNRI

(BPPV: benign paroxysmal positional vertigo; PPPD: persistent postural perceptual dizziness; SSRI: selective serotonin reuptake inhibitors; SNRI: selective noradrenergic reuptake inhibitors)

A study performed on 32 MdDS patients showed that the group that received migraine prophylactic medicines (n = 15) responded better than the group (n = 17) that received physical therapy and vestibular rehabilitation.[12]

PERSISTENT DIZZINESS AFTER MILD CONCUSSION

Concussion refers to mild traumatic brain injury with biochemical alteration rather than structural abnormalities. Concussion can lead to both central and peripheral vestibular dysfunction.

Common causes of dizziness **(Flowchart 3)** after concussion include positional vertigo, exertional dizziness, vestibular migraine, spatial disorientation, and dizziness secondary to visual disorders.

Broadly, dizziness after mild concussion usually occurs due to 2 reasons: (1)Structural abnormalities and (2) nonstructural causes.

Pathophysiology

Labyrinthine concussion following head trauma is the inciting event for postconcussion dizziness. The pathophysiology has been elucidated in **Flowchart 4**.

Time Course

Multiple factors contributing to dizziness after concussion make time course difficult to predict. Dizziness related to concussion is diagnosed by temporal profile of symptoms following an acute event. They usually recover few days after a concussion but presence of vestibulo-ocular reflex (VOR) abnormalities, migraine headaches, impending litigation, and preexisting anxiety are predictors of delayed recovery. If symptoms persist beyond 4 weeks, a term postconcussion syndrome is usually assigned.[13]

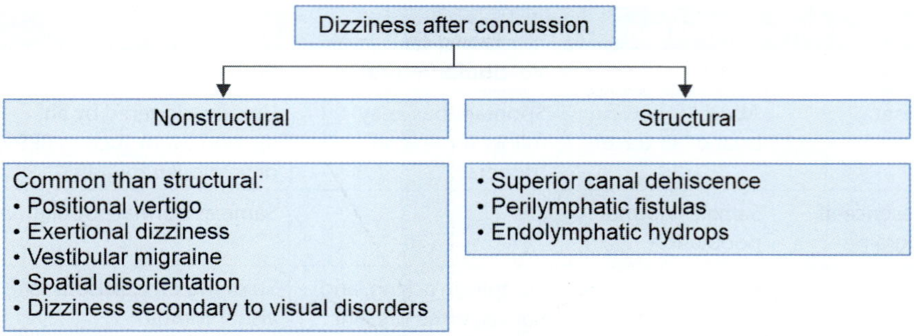

FLOWCHART 3: Causes of dizziness after concussion.[2]

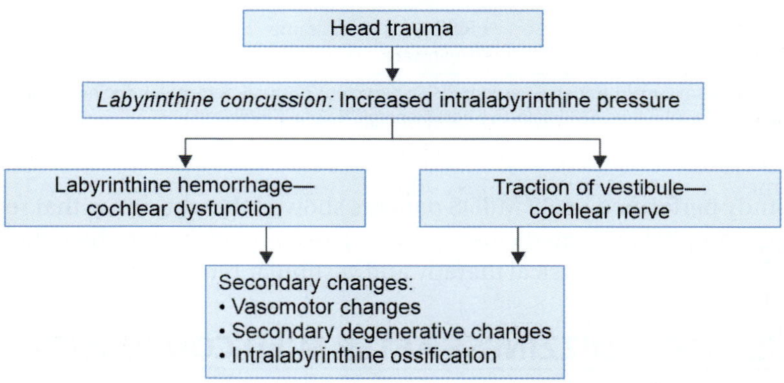

FLOWCHART 4: Pathophysiology of postconcussion dizziness.

Treatment

Functional dysfunction being more common should be addressed first. All patients have to undergo testing for benign paroxysmal positional vertigo, assessment for migraine, and screening for auditory assessment. Structural causes should be suspected when there is sound-induced dizziness and associated hearing loss.

Vestibular rehabilitation measures should be administered especially when there is VOR dysfunction. Additional symptoms may require additional management based on associated symptoms.[2]

MOTION SICKNESS

Motion sickness (aka kinetosis) was first observed as an entity by the great Greek Physician Hippocrates when he wrote that "sailing on the sea proves that motion disorders the body". The term "motion sickness" was first used by Irwin in 1881 and he noted that this occurs during repeated oscillatory movement of the body. Motion sickness usually occurs when an individual is passively transported, but occasionally it may occur in a stationary person while viewing a large moving field and during virtual reality rides in amusement parks (pseudokinetosis).[14] Thus, motion sickness may occur in various modalities of passive motion as described

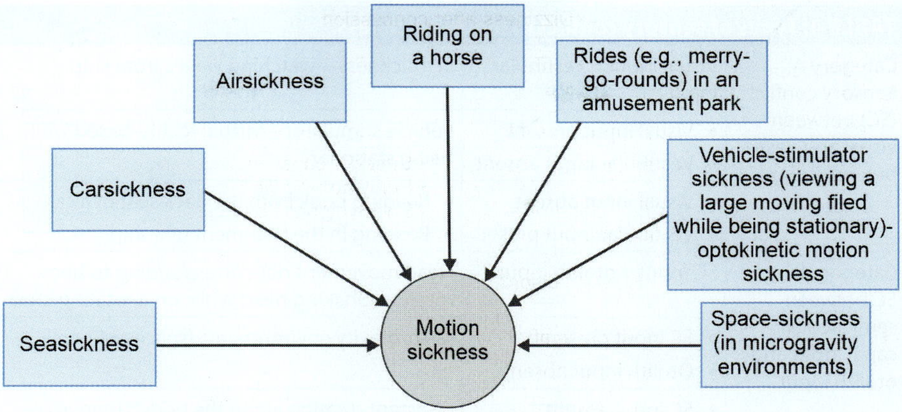

FIG. 1: Situations during which motion sickness is commonly experienced.[14]

in **Figure 1** and resistance to one type of motion may not confer resistance to other type of motion, i.e., a person who does not experience motion sickness in a flight may develop motion sickness while traveling in a car.

Pathophysiology of Motion Sickness

The percept of body posture and movement comes from three different modalities of sensory input: (1) Visual, (2) vestibular, and (3) proprioceptive inputs. These three modalities, in normal conditions, provide congruent input. Conflicts between the various sensory modalities are the current explanation for motion sickness. Incongruent sensory information from these three modalities results in conflict between visual, proprioceptive, and vestibular systems resulting in motion sickness. There are two types of sensory conflicts: (1) category A and (2) category B.[15] Category A conflict is the intersensory conflict between the vestibular and visual systems and category B conflict is the intersensory conflict between the otolith organs and the semicircular canals. Interestingly, being blind does not confer immunity against motion sickness. The various types of intersensory conflict have been described in **Table 4.**[2]

Risk groups:
- Children aged between 6–12 years
- Women
- Young adults
- People with migraine[16,17]
- Homozygous twin with motion sickness[15]
- People with Ménière's disease[18]
- Pregnant women[19]

Relatively low-risk groups:
- Children <1 year old—almost never develop motion sickness as their visual input processing is not significant enough to create conflict
- Elderly people
- People with bilateral labyrinthine disease

TABLE 4: Types of sensory conflict in motion sickness.		
Category A: Sensory conflict (SC) between visual and vestibular systems	Visual input ≠ vestibular input	Sea sickness—watching waves from ship
	• Visual input present • Vestibular input absent	Vehicle stimulator—virtual reality-based while being stationary
	• Visual input absent • Vestibular input preset	• Reading book from the back seat of a car • Reading in the basement of a ship
Category B: SC between semicircular canal input and otolith input	SC input ≠ otolith input	Head movement not corresponding to body rotation. Shaking head while on a rotating chair
	• SC input present • Otolith input absent	Microgravity environments (space sickness)
	• SC input absent • Otolith input present	Constant rotation along the body's long axis—barbeque roll

Clinical Features of Motion Sickness

Motion sickness is an acute illness with a latency from minutes to hours from stimulus onset and the resolution of symptoms occurs usually within hours to a day of cessation of the instigating stimulus. It is usually triggered by low-frequency motion, with 0.2 Hz being recorded as the frequency with the most potential for generating motion sickness. At each frequency, the occurrence of motion sickness depends further on the intensity of the stimulus; for example, floating on a raft at sea produces a much greater degree of seasickness as compared to traveling on a ship.[14] The constellation of symptoms in motion sickness can be diverse, ranging from the common nausea/vomiting, nonvertiginous lightheadedness, pallor, sweating, yawning, headache, drowsiness, loss of concentration and drive, and hypersalivation. Rarely, more incapacitating features such as postural instability, intractable retching resulting in dehydration and electrolyte losses may occur.[19] The constellation of symptoms has been described as Sopite syndrome. In certain situations such as space-travel and being a pilot in an airplane, these symptoms may be hazardous and life threatening though the term motion sickness may appear innocuous.

Nonpharmacologic Measures to Prevent Motion Sickness

Prevention of motion sickness is always easier than treating it once the symptoms have set in. Some measures can be done to avoid/mitigate the sensory conflict between visual-vestibular systems and the semicircular canal-otolith systems.

- Orienting the head in the direction of vector of the movement—facing backward in a moving vehicle will cause more severe and earlier onset of symptoms.
- Visual control of moving environment—looking at the horizon in a car, avoiding reading or watching phone during car travel. If not possible, closing the eyes is a better option.
- Orienting the head to the vector of gravitation—lying supine in a car or ship, sitting upright in a helicopter.

- Avoiding unnecessary head movements.
- Habituation—intermittent exposure to a stimulus will confer resistance to motion sickness against that particular stimulus in most individuals.
- Actively steering the vehicle.
- Listening to pleasant music and[15] controlled breathing also mitigates symptoms.[20]

Pharmacological Prevention and Treatment of Motion Sickness

Anticholinergics

Scopolamine is an anticholinergic agent effective in the prevention and treatment of motion sickness. It acts by blocking input to the vestibular nuclei and the vomiting center.[21] The various routes of administration of scopolamine and doses are given in **Table 5**.

Transdermal scopolamine is not approved for children <10 years old and it is a category-C pregnancy drug, where antihistaminic diphenhydramine is preferred. Scopolamine is also not to be used by those involved in driving or heavy machinery work. It is contraindicated in patients with glaucoma and prostatic enlargement.

Antihistaminic Agents

First-generation sedating antihistaminic agents (diphenhydramine, dimenhydrinate, cinnarizine, cyclizine, meclizine, and promethazine) are useful in preventing and treating motion sickness, whereas second generation nonsedating antihistaminic agents (cetirizine, fexofenadine, and loratadine) are not useful in preventing or treating motion sickness.[22] These agents antagonize histamine receptors in the vomiting center and also have anticholinergic activity. Their onset of action is delayed as compared to scopolamine and has to be taken orally at least 2 hours prior to the intended travel. These drugs are more sedating than scopolamine. These agents may be used in combination with sympathomimetics (ephedrine or dextroamphetamine), which serve to counteract their sedating effects. Common dosages are given as follows:

- Dimenhydrinate 100 mg oral
- Promethazine 25 mg with or without amphetamine 25 mg

TABLE 5: Doses of scopolamine and routes of administration.

Route	Application site and time of application	Dose and duration of action	Adverse events
Transdermal patch	• Mastoid process • 4–8 hours prior to intended travel	• 0.5–1 mg patch • Works for 72 hours	Dry mouth, dry eyes, blurred vision, confusion, headache, drowsiness, acute angle, closure glaucoma, restlessness, and memory
Oral	30 minutes to 1 hour prior to travel	• 0.3–0.6 mg • Works for 4–6 hours	
Parenteral	Intramuscular (IM) injection	0.3–0.6 mg stat	
	Can be given even after nausea and vomiting have set in		Disturbances and hallucination

Meclizine and diphenhydramine are pregnancy category-B drugs and are used more commonly in pregnant patients. Scopolamine and promethazine are pregnancy category-C drugs.

Complementary and alternative medicines:
- Using ginger candies is effective though their exact mechanism of action is unclear. In a blind placebo-controlled study, powdered rhizomes of ginger (940 mg in gelatin capsule) were compared with 100 mg dimenhydrinate, and ginger was found to be more effective than dimenhydrinate.[23]
- Acupressure or acupuncture at the P2 point (anterior surface of forearm, 2 inches proximal to the distal wrist crease, between the middle two tendons) is said to be useful in preventing and treating motion sickness.[24,25]

BILATERAL VESTIBULOPATHY

Bilateral vestibulopathy (BVP), previously known by the name Dandy syndrome, is a common, likely underdiagnosed disease of primarily the elderly population. It is a consequence of the loss of sensory input from the vestibular system, which leads as a result of damage in any part of the pathway from the vestibular end organs to the vestibular nucleus in the brainstem—semicircular canals and otolith organs, vestibular nerve, vestibular nerve root entry zone, and vestibular nucleus in the brainstem. Thus, the affected person utilizes the visual system and the proprioceptive system to compensate for the loss of input from the vestibular system. The reported prevalence ranges from 28–81 per lakh population and it is likely an underestimation of the burden of the problem.[26]

Pathophysiology

The vestibular system has two main effector areas—(1) the ocular motor system and (2) the spinal cord, via the vestibulo-ocular pathways and the vestibulospinal pathways. The vestibulo-ocular system serves to stabilize ocular fixation during head movements so that the object of interest remains on the fovea. Dysfunction of this system results in slipping of the object of interest from the fovea during eye movements, resulting in blurring and oscillopsia during head movements. The vestibulospinal system involves the vestibulospinal tract, which is important for maintenance of the upright posture. Thus, dysfunction of the vestibular system produces a sense of significant imbalance only when standing or walking and not while lying down/sitting.[27] The pathophysiological basis of symptoms in bilateral vestibulopathy is mentioned in **Flowchart 5**.

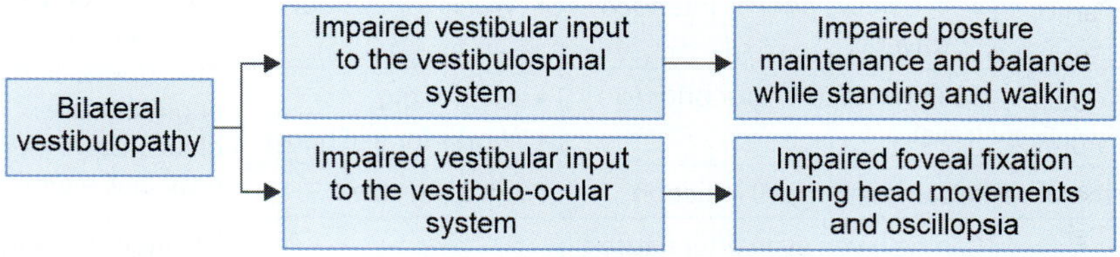

FLOWCHART 5: Basis of various symptoms in bilateral vestibulopathy.

Etiology

Multiple etiological factors are causative for BVP, the most common being ototoxic drugs, genetic disorders, and the meningitis. In some conditions, central causes of ataxia and sensory ataxia can coexist—cerebellar ataxia with neuropathy and vestibular areflexia syndrome (CANVAS), SCA27B, SCA3, SCA6. Some of the etiologic causes of BVP are given in the **Box 3**.

Clinical Features

History

The characteristic clinical feature of BVP is a sense of dizziness and postural imbalance while walking and standing, which worsens in the dark and while on uneven ground. The patients do not have any symptoms in static conditions while lying or sitting. Additionally, they also complain of blurring of vision or oscillopsia, while walking or running. The patients find it difficult to read road signposts while walking or in a vehicle. Blurring can also occur on fast head turns to either side, but not during slow head turns as the pursuit system is able to compensate and maintain foveal fixation. Spinning vertigo is not a characteristic feature in BVP as it reflects asymmetry of vestibular function. However, presence of spinning vertigo during the early stages of disease may point to certain

BOX 3 Etiologies of bilateral vestibulopathy.

- Genetic:
  - DFNA9, DFNA11, DFNA15, and DFNB4
- Infectious:
  - Meningitis
  - HSV vestibular neuritis
  - Syphilis
  - Lyme disease
  - Rubella
  - Herpes zoster
- Drug-induced vestibulopathy:
  - Chemotherapy—cisplatin
  - Aminoglycosides
  - Furosemide
  - Immune checkpoint inhibitors
  - Amiodarone
  - NSAIDs and penicillin
- Inflammatory:
  - Susac syndrome
  - Cogan's syndrome
  - Autoimmune inner ear disease
  - Sarcoidosis
  - Behçet's disease
  - Celiac disease
- Tumors:
  - Vestibular
  - Schwannoma
  - Neurofibromatosis 2
  - Metastasis
  - Lymphoma
- Neurodegenerative:
  - SCA 27B, SCA 3, and SCA 6
  - Friedreich's ataxia
  - CANVAS
- Others:
  - Superficial siderosis
  - Vitamin B_{12} and folate deficiency
  - Superficial siderosis
  - Vestibular migraine
  - Wernicke's encephalopathy

etiologies—autoimmune etiology and Méniére's disease. In some diseases, cerebellar ataxia and neuropathy may also coexist as in SCA 27B and CANVAS.[28] Presence of bilateral progressive hypoacusis may indicate bilateral schwannoma. Gait is affected and though partially compensated by sensory reweighting (over reliance on visual and proprioceptive information), signs such as increased cadence and broad-based walking are evident. Additionally, there is significant worsening when the compensatory mechanism is disturbed—as in walking in a dimly lit environment.

Physical Examination

While examining a patient with suspected BVP, it is necessary to test for cerebellar function (finger-nose-finger test, heel-shin test, and dysdiadochokinesia) and disorders of proprioception (Romberg test, tandem Romberg test, and sensory examination especially for vibration and position sense). The key tests that have to be performed in a patient with suspected BVP have been described as follows:

- *Head impulse test (HIT):* It detects severe BVP. It is sufficiently sensitive only when performed by an experienced examiner and if VOR gain is <0.4. False negatives may occur due to covert saccades, inexperienced examiner, and in mild BVP.
- *Visually-assisted vestibulo-ocular reflex (VVOR):* It picks up a combination of vestibular and cerebellar involvement. The patient is asked to fix on a stationary object (e.g., examiner's nose) and his/her head is slowly turned from side-to-side. Presence of broken, saccadic pursuits indicates dysfunction.[26]
- Dynamic visual acuity is a complementary test, which may be done by testing the visual acuity while walking on a treadmill.

Laboratory Tests

The investigatory modalities that are helpful in establishing a diagnosis of BVP, which are incorporated in the Barany criteria are:

- *Video nystagmography (v-HIT) or scleral coil technique to measure VOR gain:* Bilateral horizontal angular VOR gain < 0.6 indicates BVP
- *Caloric stimulation test:* A reduced caloric response (sum of bithermal maximum peak slow phase velocity (SPV) < 6°/second)
- *Rotatory chair testing:* Reduced horizontal angular VOR gain < 0.1 upon sinusoidal stimulation and a phase lead >68° (tie constant < 5 seconds)

Other investigatory modalities that may be helpful but not a part of the Barany criteria are:

- Testing of oscillopsia by functional HIT (fHIT test)
- Cervical and ocular vestibular evoked myogenic potentials (c-VEMP and o-VEMP)

Diagnostic Criteria

Barany society had proposed the diagnostic criteria for BVP in 2017. The diagnosis of definite BVP requires abnormality in at least one of the three investigatory modalities mentioned earlier and in the absence of laboratory assistance, a

TABLE 6: Bárány Society criteria for bilateral vestibulopathy (BVP).[29]		
Definite BVP	A. Chronic vestibular syndrome with the following symptoms	Unsteadiness while walking or standing + at least one of the following: 1. Movement-induced blurring of vision or oscillopsia while walking or during quick head/body movements 2. Worsening of unsteadiness in darkness and/or on uneven ground
	B. No symptoms while sitting or lying down under static conditions	
	C. Bilaterally reduced or absent angular vestibulo-ocular reflex (VOR) function as documented by	1. Video-nystagmography (v-HIT) or scleral coil technique to measure VOR gain; bilateral horizontal angular VOR gain < 0.6 indicates BVP and/or 2. *Caloric stimulation test*: A reduced caloric response [sum of bithermal maximum peak slow phase velocity (SPV) < 6°/second] and/or 3. *Rotatory chair testing*: Reduced horizontal angular VOR gain <0.1 upon sinusoidal stimulation and a phase lead > 68° (tie constant < 5 seconds)
	D. Not better accounted by another disease	
Probable BVP	A. Chronic vestibular syndrome with the following symptoms	Unsteadiness while walking or standing + at least one of the following: 1. Movement-induced blurring of vision or oscillopsia while walking or during quick head/body movements 2. Worsening of unsteadiness in darkness and/or on uneven ground
	B. No symptoms while sitting or lying down under static conditions	
	C. Bilaterally abnormal bedside horizontal head impulse test	
	D. Not better accounted by another disease	

diagnosis of probable BVP can be made based on the bedside findings. The Bárány Society criteria have been described in **Table 6**.

Management

The management of patients with BVP includes the following:

- Communicating to the patients about the nature of their disease
- Vestibular rehabilitation exercises
- Arresting progressive damage, if possible
- Recovery of lost vestibular function, if possible

Communicating to Patients about Nature of Their Disease

The diagnosis of BVP is often delayed, and the patient is more likely to have visited multiple clinics without appropriate diagnosis. This serves to intensify the patient's symptoms and anxiety. Explaining to the patients about the nature of disease, possible mechanisms, and the plan of management will serve to establish rapport and will prepare the patient for adhering to the subsequent treatment plan. Management of patients with BVP requires vestibular rehabilitation exercises over long periods, which have to be done daily and knowledge about the disease will help make compliance easier.

Vestibular Rehabilitation Exercises

Physical rehabilitation exercises work on the principle of (1) adaptation or (2) substitution. Exercises involving adaptation strategy aim to maximize the gain of the residual function of the vestibular system. Substitutive strategies act to use the alternate modalities of sensory input (visual and proprioception) to compensate for the loss of function of the vestibular system. Though substitution measures are helpful, it is not possible to entirely compensate for the magnitude of deficits caused by dysfunction of the vestibular system. For example, somatosensory system is unable to generate as fast a response as the VOR system and vestibulospinal system. As a result, a patient with BVP is less capable of reacting reflexively to postural challenges despite rehabilitation measures.[26] Postural disturbances take longer to recover as compared to gaze-stability disturbances. Some of the vestibular rehabilitation strategies are given in **Table 1**.

Arresting Progressive Damage

Prevention of further insults causing vestibular damage is especially relevant in vestibulopathy due to ototoxic drug use. Aminoglycosides should be used only if necessary, and if used, once daily dosing is preferred. Concurrent use of ototoxic drugs, such a furosemide, and nonsteroidal anti-inflammatory drugs (NSAIDs) should be avoided. It is important to note that aminoglycoside-induced vestibulopathy may occur days or weeks after exposure to the drug.[28]

Recovery of Lost Vestibular Function

Vestibular dysfunction may be due to treatable causes such as infection (meningitis, cholesteatoma, herpes simplex virus (HSV) vestibular neuritis, Lyme's disease, and syphilis) or autoimmune conditions (Cogan's syndrome, autoimmune inner ear disease, Sjögren syndrome, Susac's syndrome, and sarcoidosis). In patients with systemic features and strong clinical suspicion of autoimmune disease, it may be expedient to start high-dose glucocorticoids (80 mg/day to be tapered over 3–4 weeks). In some conditions such as Cogan's syndrome, pulse dose of methylprednisolone 1 g/day IV for 5 days is also advisable. Treating nutritional deficiencies (thiamine, vitamin B_{12}, and folate) is also indicated.[28]

Finally, vestibular implants have been studied and were found to improve gait stability. They are more effective in patients with residual vestibular function. These devices appear to meet the expectation of patients with respect to functional improvements and are very promising.[30]

CONCLUSION

This article attempts to summarize various causes of persistent dizziness. Many conditions which were previously termed functional dizziness have been re-classified here. Recognition of many of these disorders and addressing them via appropriate drugs or vestibular rehabilitation helps mitigate term disability.

REFERENCES

1. Cha YH. Chronic dizziness. CONTINUUM: Lifelong Learning in Neurology. 2021;27(2):420-46.
2. Knight B, Bermudez F, Shermetaro C. Persistent postural–perceptual dizziness. In: StatPearls [Internet]. Treasure Island (FL): StatPearls Publishing; 2025. Available from https://www.ncbi.nlm.nih.gov/books/NBK578198/ [Last accessed April, 2025].
3. Staab JP, Eckhardt-Henn A, Bronstein A, Horii A, Jacob R, Strupp M, et al. Diagnostic criteria for persistent postural-perceptual dizziness (PPPD): Consensus document of the committee for the Classification of Vestibular Disorders of the Bárány Society. J Vestib Res. 2017;27(4).
4. Han BI, Song HS, Kim JS. Vestibular rehabilitation therapy: Review of indications, mechanisms, and key exercises. J Clin Neurol. 2011;7(4):184-96.
5. Han BI, Han BI. Vestibular rehabilitation therapy: Review of indications, mechanisms, and key exercises. J Clin Neurol. 2011;7(4):184-96.
6. Axer H, Finn S, Wassermann A, Guntinas-Lichius O, Klingner CM, Witte OW. Multimodal treatment of persistent postural–perceptual dizziness. Brain Behav. 2020;10(12):e01864.
7. Zang J, Zheng M, Chu H, Yang X. Additional cognitive behavior therapy for persistent postural–perceptual dizziness: A meta-analysis. Braz J Otorhinolaryngol. 2024;90(3):101393.
8. Webster KE, Harrington-Benton NA, Judd O, Kaski D, Maarsingh OR, MacKeith S, et al. Pharmacological interventions for persistent postural-perceptual dizziness (PPPD). Cochrane Database Syst Rev. 2023;3(3):CD015188.
9. Neurology Department, University of Utah Health. (2023). Medication management for PPPD. [online]. Available from https://medicine.utah.edu/neurology/education/dizzy-school/pppd/medication-management [Last accessed April, 2025].
10. Cha YH, Baloh RW, Cho C, Magnusson M, Song JJ, Strupp M, et al. Mal de débarquement syndrome diagnostic criteria: Consensus document of the Classification Committee of the Bárány Society. J Vestib Res. 2020;30(5):285-93.
11. Saha KC, Fife TD. Mal de débarquement syndrome: Review and proposed diagnostic criteria. Neurol Clin Pract. 2015;5(3):209-15.
12. Ghavami Y, Ziai KN, Haidar YM, Moshtaghi O, Bhatt J, Lin HW, et al. Management of mal de debarquement syndrome as vestibular migraines. Laryngoscope. 2016;127(7):1670-5.
13. Gianoli GJ. Post-concussive dizziness: A review and clinical approach to the patient. Front Neurol. 2022;12:718318.
14. Leung AK, Hon KL. Motion sickness: An overview. Drugs in context. 2019;8:2019-9-4.
15. Koch A, Cascorbi I, Westhofen M, Dafotakis M, Klapa S, Kuhtz-Buschbeck JP. The neurophysiology and treatment of motion sickness. Dtsch Arztebl Int. 2018;115(41):687.
16. Granston A, Drummond PD. Migraine and motion sickness: What is the link? Prog Neurobiol. 2010;91(4):300-12.
17. Drummond PD. Triggers of motion sickness in migraine sufferers. Headache. 2005;45(6):653-6.
18. Golding JF, Patel M. Meniere's, migraine, and motion sickness. Acta Otolaryngol. 2017;137(5):495-502.
19. Takov V, Tadi P. Motion Sickness. In: StatPearls [Internet]. Treasure Island (FL): StatPearls Publishing; 2024. Available from https://www.ncbi.nlm.nih.gov/books/NBK539706/ [Last accessed April, 2025].
20. Jokerst MD, Gatto M, Fazio R, Stern RM, Koch KL. Slow deep breathing prevents the development of tachygastria and symptoms of motion sickness. Aviat Space Environ Med. 1999;70(12):1189-92.
21. Schmäl F. Neuronal mechanisms and the treatment of motion sickness. Pharmacology. 2013;91(3-4):229-41.
22. Cheung BS, Heskin R, Hofer KD. Failure of cetirizine and fexofenadine to prevent motion sickness. Ann Pharmacother. 2003;37(2):173-7.
23. Mowrey DB, Clayson DE. Motion sickness, ginger, and psychophysics. Lancet. 1982;1(8273):655-7.
24. Hu S, Stritzel R, Chandler A, Stern RM. P6 acupressure reduces symptoms of vection-induced motion sickness. Aviat Space Environ Med. 1995;66(7):631-4.

25. Stern RM, Jokerst MD, Muth ER, Hollis C. Acupressure relieves the symptoms of motion sickness and reduces abnormal gastric activity. Altern Ther Health Med. 2001;7(4):91-4.
26. van Stiphout L, Szmulewicz DJ, Guinand N, Fornos AP, Van Rompaey V, van de Berg R. Bilateral vestibulopathy: A clinical update and proposed diagnostic algorithm. Front Neurol. 2023;14:1308485.
27. Yoo H, Mihaila DM. Neuroanatomy, Vestibular Pathways. In: StatPearls [Internet]. Treasure Island (FL): StatPearls Publishing; 2024 . Available from https://www.ncbi.nlm.nih.gov/books/NBK557380/ [Last accessed April, 2025]
28. Strupp M, Feil K, Dieterich M, Brandt T. Bilateral vestibulopathy. Handb Clin Neurol. 2016;137:235-40.
29. Strupp M, Kim JS, Murofushi T, Straumann D, Jen JC, Rosengren SM, et al. Bilateral vestibulopathy: Diagnostic criteria Consensus document of the Classification Committee of the Bárány Society. J Vestib Res. 2017;27(4):177-89.
30. Starkov D, Guinand N, Lucieer F, Ranieri M, Cavuscens S, Pleshkov M, et al. Restoring the high-frequency dynamic visual acuity with a vestibular implant prototype in humans. Audiol Neuro-otol. 2020;25(1-2):91-5.

10

CHAPTER

Central Vertigo

Philo Hazeena, Nelabhotla Sai Satya Saranya

ABSTRACT

Central vertigo represents a heterogeneous group of disorders resulting from dysfunctions in the central vestibular pathways including the brainstem, cerebellum, thalamus and cortex. It accounts for 25% of vertigo cases and often mimics peripheral vestibulopathies leading to diagnostic challenges. A detailed understanding of characteristic oculomotor signs and the application of integrated clinical, laboratory and imaging approaches are critical for accurate diagnosis and management of central vertigo.

INTRODUCTION

Central vertigo is a false sensation of motion caused by a lesion in the central nervous system (CNS) that results in dysfunction of the vestibular nuclei or their projections to the cerebellum. Vestibular illnesses are categorized according to the anatomical location into central and peripheral vertigo. The components of the vestibular system are posture, gait, spatial orientation, ocular motor control, and perception of body position and motion.

Central disorders are diseases pertaining to the vestibular nuclei within the pontomedullary brainstem and the vestibular pathways that project from these nuclei to the vestibulocerebellum (via the cerebellar peduncles), brainstem, thalamus, and cortex.

Dizziness and vertigo are common complaints in neurology, where 25% of patients tend to have a central origin, 32% have a peripheral vestibular cause in addition to functional (somatoform) and psychiatric causes which comprise about 18% of vertigo and dizziness cases.[1-3]

Central vertigo requires early diagnosis and prompt treatment, given its grave prognosis.

CENTRAL VESTIBULAR SYSTEM (FLOWCHART 1 AND FIG. 1)

The functions can be separated into four anatomically distinct groups:

1. Control of balance
2. Gaze control during head and body movements
3. Perception of orientation and self-motion and integration of voluntary motion with reflexive motion and balance control, mediated at cortical and subcortical levels.
4. Higher vestibular functions involving multisensory integration and cognitive domains such as spatial memory and navigation, are mediated mainly by the hippocampal formation and the temporoparietal lobes.[4]

The most important structures are the neuronal pathways mediating the vestibulo-ocular reflex (VOR).

They travel from the peripheral labyrinth over the vestibular nuclei in the medullary brainstem to the ocular motor nuclei (III, IV, and VI) and the supranuclear integration centers in the pons and midbrain (interstitial nucleus

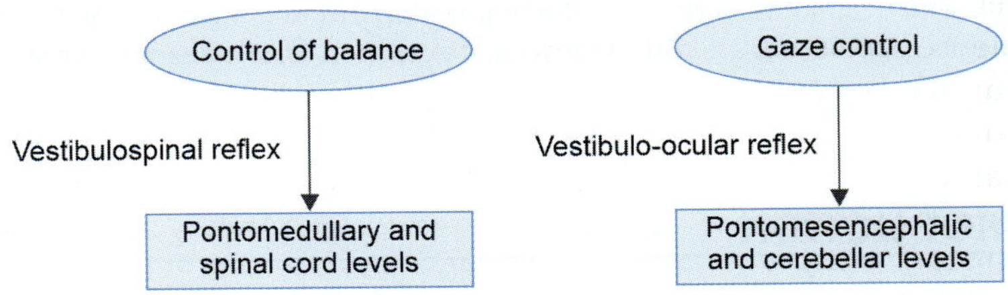

FLOWCHART 1: Vestibular functions.[5]

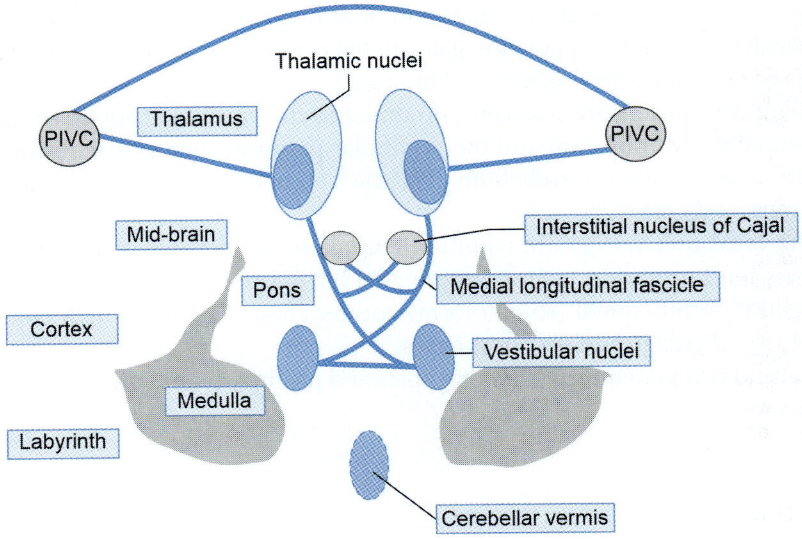

FIG. 1: Central vestibular system.[5]

of Cajal INC and rostral interstitial nucleus of the medial longitudinal fascicle, riMLF). Ascending pathways travel contralaterally and ipsilaterally over the posterolateral thalamus up to a network of vestibular areas in the parietotemporal cortex and the insula parietoinsular vestibular cortex (PIVC), areas in the superior temporal gyrus, and inferior parietal lobes, which are responsible for perception. Descending pathways lead from the vestibular nuclei along the medial and lateral vestibulospinal tract into the spinal cord to mediate postural control.[5]

To produce a global perception and sufficient motor responses to the actual sensory input, the bilateral organization of the vestibular system necessitates a constant interaction between the right and left circuits at all levels, particularly between the two hemispheres. This allows balance to be maintained within the gravitational field. In the event of acute unilateral impairment, bilateral representation of vestibular functions permits the replacement of unilaterally damaged pathways and serves as the foundation for central compensation of a tone imbalance.[6,7]

ETIOLOGY (FLOWCHART 2)

The three clinical manifestations of central vertigo **(Box 1)**:

1. Acute attacks of vertigo and dizziness
2. Recurrent attacks
3. Chronic central vertigo

In patients with acute onset, it is essential to differentiate between central and peripheral vertigo because this has major diagnostic and therapeutic implications.

A differentiation can most often be achieved by a careful neuro-ophthalmological and neuro-otological bedside examination.

Short rotatory or postural vertigo attacks lasting seconds to minutes or few hours	• Transient ischemic attacks within vertibrobasilar artery • Vestibular migraine • Paroxysmal brainstem attacks with ataxia/dysarthria in MS, vestibular epilepsy
Attacks of rotatory or postural vertigo lasting hours to several days with additional brainstem defects	• Infarction, hemorrhage, cavernoma, tumors or MS plaques in the brainstem and/or vestibulocerebellum • Long lasting attacks of vestibular migraine
Persisting postural imbalace and dizziness, combined with tendency to fall	• Permanent damage to brainstem or cerebellum bilaterally • Downbeat nystagmus syndrome due to flocculus/paraflocculus dysfunction • Transient upbeat syndrome due to paramedian pontomedullary or pontomesencephalic damage

FLOWCHART 2: Etiology of central vertigo.[20]

(MS: multiple sclerosis)

BOX 1 Clinical signs of central vertigo.[20]

- Skew deviation/vertical divergence (as part of the ocular tilt reaction)
- Gaze-evoked nystagmus contralateral to a spontaneous nystagmus
- Saccadic smooth pursuit
- Nonpathological head-impulse test in patients with an acute nystagmus
- Central fixation nystagmus (which contrary to peripheral vestibular spontaneous nystagmus is not suppressed by visual fixation)

The five signs indicating of central lesions:

This 5-step procedure has a sensitivity of >95% for evidence of a central lesion; this sensitivity is higher than that possible with early magnetic resonance imaging (MRI) with diffusion-weighted sequences (88%).[8,9]

CENTRAL NERVOUS SYSTEM CAUSES OF VERTIGO

Vestibular Migraine (Box 2)

Vestibular migraine is the most common form of episodic vertigo and affects both children and adults. This accounts for 7–11% of outpatients seen in dizziness units and 9% of outpatients seen in migraine units. Women are affected 1.5–5.0 times more often than men.

International Headache Society and the International Bárány Society for Neuro-otology accepted the term "vestibular migraine" and have developed diagnostic criteria for vestibular migraine.[10,11]

Vestibular migraine causes episodic vertigo that can appear positional, spontaneously, or visually induced. Vestibular symptoms may occur during headaches but also commonly occur without headaches. Between episodes, patients may experience chronic dizziness and imbalance. Vertigo can precede, accompany, or even follow the headache. The attack can last from seconds to days but is most frequently in the range of minutes to hours. Central ocular motor dysfunctions, such as gaze-evoked nystagmus, pursuit deficits, central positional nystagmus, and dysmetria or slow saccades can be noted on examination.[12,13]

In 30% of patients with vestibular migraine typical migraine headache is absent, spontaneous vertigo is seen in 21–83% of attacks, positional vertigo or dizziness in 17–65% of attacks, and head motion intolerance and postural imbalance in 31–77% of attacks.[12,14,15]

The differential diagnosis of vestibular migraine are the early stage of Ménière endolymphatic hydrops when aural symptoms are absent and episodic ataxia type 2 (EA2).

Multiple Sclerosis

Multiple sclerosis (MS) causes inflammatory demyelinating lesions throughout the CNS and is known to cause lesions specifically in areas that result in vertigo (i.e., the brainstem and cerebellum). 20% of patients with MS will experience true vertigo, and in about 5% of patients with MS, it is the presenting symptom of the disease. The most common CNS sites known to cause vertigo in MS are lesions at

BOX 2 Diagnostic criteria for vestibular migraine.[5,10]

- At least five episodes fulfilling criteria C and D below
- A current or past history of migraine without aura or migraine with aura
- Vestibular symptoms of moderate or severe intensity, lasting 5 minutes to 72 hours
- At least 50% of episodes are associated with at least one of the following three migrainous features:
    i. Headache with at least two of the following four characteristics: (1) unilateral location, (2) pulsating quality, (3) moderate or severe intensity, (4) aggravation by routine physical activity
    ii. Photophobia and phonophobia
    iii. Visual aura
- Not better accounted for by another diagnosis from the third edition of the International Classification of Headache Disorders, or by another vestibular disorder

the root entry zone of cranial nerve VIII (the lateral pontomedullary junction) and the medial vestibular nucleus.[16]

Vertigo due to MS may present acutely during an exacerbation, or it can persist in a chronic form as a result of disease burden. During an exacerbation, vertigo can be accompanied by nausea and vomiting. Patients may be ataxic and may also report diplopia.

Central vertigo from MS is usually seen along with various focal findings on neurologic examination. Abnormal saccades with reduced velocities, nystagmus (potentially in multiple directions), impaired suppression of the vestibulo-ocular reflex, and internuclear ophthalmoplegia (INO) are the prominent features that can be observed. INO is the most common eye movement disorder seen in MS and is caused by demyelination of the medial longitudinal fasciculus in the pons or midbrain. Patients with MS may have saccadic dysmetria from cerebellar involvement, particularly when the cerebellar peduncle is affected. Cerebellar lesions can also cause impaired smooth pursuit and gaze-evoked, downbeat, or acquired pendular nystagmus that may be associated with oculopalatal tremors and often with dizziness, imbalance, and oscillopsia (a perception of objects bouncing or oscillating). Acquired pendular nystagmus likely results from damage to the neural integrator network in the brainstem and cerebellum.[16,17]

Stroke and Transient Ischemic Attack

Strokes and transient ischemic attacks (TIAs) are known causes of central vertigo, dizziness, and imbalance when the posterior circulation is affected. Cerebellar ischemic stroke in the posterior inferior cerebellar artery (PICA) territory, the anterior inferior cerebellar artery (AICA) territory, or the superior cerebellar artery territory may be associated with vertigo or nystagmus, or both.

Vertigo and nystagmus commonly occur when the area of infarction affects the cerebellar peduncles, flocculus, nodulus, vermis, and paravermian regions and are less common with small lesions that are far lateral in the cerebellar hemisphere. Vertigo may also manifest from a brainstem infarction, which can affect the lateral medulla, medial medulla, pons, or midbrain. Vertigo with unilateral hearing loss can be caused by a labyrinthine infarction. The labyrinth is supplied by the internal auditory artery, usually a branch of the AICA. Chronic vertigo due to the late effects of stroke is not an uncommon symptom; it is often a residual symptom that can persist long after the infarct occurs.[18,19]

Tumors and Other Structural Lesions in Central Nervous System

Neoplasms and vascular lesions cause central vertigo and other neurologic symptoms based on their location in the CNS, including vestibular schwannoma, cavernous malformation, hemangioblastoma, and medulloblastoma.

Vertigo is an infrequent presentation of vestibular schwannoma, estimated which is seen in <15% of patients. Slowly progressive unilateral hearing loss and tinnitus are more common initial symptoms. When patients present with dizziness, they may be described as spinning vertigo, lightheadedness, or gait imbalance. As vestibular schwannomas enlarge, they may lead to peripheral vestibular loss and can lead to loss of balance. These tumors can also grow to compress the brainstem and thereby cause central vertigo.

Hemangioblastoma can cause vertigo and ataxia because of compression of structures in the brainstem or cerebellum or because of hemorrhage in those areas. In the cerebellum, where they are usually present, these often appear as enhancing nodules within a cyst.

Medulloblastoma is the most common malignant brain tumor diagnosed in children. It presents with headache, nausea, and vomiting, often because of fourth ventricle involvement causing increased intracranial pressure. In addition, patients may present with vertigo due to brainstem compression and cerebellar involvements.[21]

Neurodegenerative Diseases

Vertigo and dizziness are commonly seen in patients with Parkinson's disease, multiple system atrophy, progressive supranuclear palsy, and cerebellar ataxia. Cerebellar ataxia has numerous potential etiologies, such as genetic disease, vitamin deficiencies, paraneoplastic disease, environmental/toxin exposures, and as a result of adverse effects of medications.

Vertigo is often paroxysmal, and bedside examination usually reveals central nystagmus. Typical patterns include spontaneous downbeat nystagmus and direction-changing horizontal end-gaze nystagmus. Downbeat nystagmus results from degeneration of the cerebellum, leading to floccular hypofunction.[21]

Episodic Ataxias

Seven autosomal dominant episodic ataxias have been identified, named episodic ataxia type 1 through episodic ataxia type 7. Of these types, most cases encountered are usually episodic ataxia type 1 or episodic ataxia type 2.

In patients with episodic ataxia type 2, vertigo is severe and episodic, accompanied by nausea, vomiting, and unsteadiness. Patients with episodic ataxia type 2 usually start having episodes during adolescence, and each episode can last hours. Stress is a common trigger, as are heat, exertion, alcohol, and caffeine. Genetic testing usually reveals mutations in the *CACNA1A* gene, specifically in the P/Q-type calcium channel α1A subunit.

Episodic ataxia type 2 is felt to be caused by a loss of P/Q-type calcium channel function in the cerebellum, in both Purkinje cells and granule layer neurons.

On neurological examination, patients often have a central pattern of nystagmus not only during their episodes but even between episodes.[19]

Toxic and Metabolic Causes

Vertigo and dizziness are common symptoms of heat illness. Loss of Purkinje cells and cerebellar atrophy in patients with heat stroke suggest vestibulocerebellar dysfunction as a common mechanism of delayed vestibulopathy after heat exposure.

Drugs like metronidazole can cause cerebellar dysfunction. The radiological imaging in metronidazole toxicity showed cerebellar lesions involving deep cerebellar nuclei. These findings may be ascribed to central or central with peripheral vestibulopathy. Pregabalin may also cause reversible vertigo.[19]

CENTRAL VESTIBULAR SYNDROMES AND DISORDERS OF HIGHER VESTIBULAR FUNCTION (TABLE 1)

These are the list of the disorders that are linked to the central lesions at multiple levels presenting as cortical, thalamic, brainstem, or cerebellar lesions.[5]

MANANGEMENT

Vestibular Migraine

The medications used in prophylaxis are flunarizine, propranolol, and venlafaxine. These drugs significantly reduce the frequency and severity of vertigo.

TABLE 1: Central vestibular syndromes and disorders of higher vestibular function.[5]

Vestibular cortex	Vestibular thalamus	Brainstem	Cerebellum
• Cortical vertigo • Pusher syndrome • Room tilt illusion • Spatial hemineglect • Spatial memory deficit • Vestibular epilepsy	• Thalamic astasia • Pusher syndrome	• Lateropulsion • Ocular tilt reaction • Paroxysmal ataxia/ dysarthria • Pseudoneuritis • Room tilt illusion • Skew–torsion • Vestibular migraine	• Downbeat nystagmus • Episodic ataxia type 2 • Ocular tilt reaction • Positional vertigo/ nystagmus • Pseudoneuritis • Upbeat nystagmus

Multiple Sclerosis

Acute attacks usually consist of corticosteroids for most MS patients who are able to tolerate them. Vestibular therapy is not usually of strong benefit for central vertigo in MS. It has been shown to improve balance and disability due to dizziness or general disequilibrium.[19]

Treatment of eye movement dysfunction is both pharmacological and nonpharmacological.

PHARMACOLOGICAL

- Acquired pendular nystagmus-gabapentin and memantine.
- Downbeat nystagmus—clonazepam, baclofen, or gabapentin in some patients with MS.
- *Vertical nystagmus and central positional nystagmus*: Dalfampridine.

NONPHARMACOLOGICAL TREATMENT

Prism lenses can be helpful for some types of nystagmus and diplopia. Improvement in nystagmus does not always result in improvement in the symptoms of dizziness or unsteadiness, but it can lessen oscillopsia for some.

Symptomatic Management

Vertigo can be managed with antiemetics or vestibular suppressants, such as benzodiazepine. Therapy programs with visual-vestibular stimulation during therapy can result in greater improvements in patients with stroke.

CONCLUSION

The process of determining whether vertigo has a central etiology begins with meticulous history taking followed by a detailed examination with particular attention to eye movements, coordination, gait, and speech. Careful examination skills are paramount in diagnosing central vertigo, as brain imaging has limitations in certain etiologies. A variety of treatments ranging from medications and visual-vestibular stimulation therapies to even surgical interventions may be employed to treat central vertigo.

REFERENCES

1. Vanni S, Nazerian P, Casati C, Moroni F, Risso M, Ottaviani M, et al. Can emergency physicians accurately and reliably assess acute vertigo in the emergency department? Emerg Med Australas. 2015;27(2):126-31.
2. Kerber KA. Vertigo and dizziness in the emergency department. Emerg Med Clin North Am. 2009;27(1):39-50.
3. Cnyrim CD, Newman-Toker D, Karch C, Brandt T, Strupp M. Normal head impulse test differentiates acute cerebellar strokes from vestibular neuritis. J Neurol Neurosurg Psychiatry. 2008;79(4):458-60.

4. Dieterich M, Brandt T. The bilateral central vestibular system: its pathways, functions, and disorders. Ann NY Acad Sci. 2015;1343:10-26.
5. Brandt T, Dieterich M. The dizzy patient: don't forget disorders of the central vestibular system. Nat Rev Neurol. 2017;13(6):352-62.
6. Straka H, Vibert N, Vidal PP, Moore LE, Dutia MB. Intrinsic membrane properties of vertebrate vestibular neurons: function, development, and plasticity. Prog Neurobiol. 2005;76(6): 349-92.
7. CCullen KE, Minor LB, Beraneck M, Sadeghi SG. Neural substrates underlying vestibular compensation: contribution of peripheral versus central processing. J Vestib Res. 2009;19 (5-6):171-82.
8. Kattah JC, Talkad AV, Wang DZ, Hsieh YH, Newman-Toker DE. HINTS to diagnose stroke in the acute vestibular syndrome: Three-step bedside oculomotor examination more sensitive than early MRI diffusion-weighted imaging. Stroke. 2009;40(11):3504-10.
9. Thompson TL, Amedee R. Vertigo: a review of common peripheral and central vestibular disorders. Ochsner J. 2009 Spring;9(1):20-6.
10. Dieterich M, Brandt T. Episodic vertigo related to migraine (90 cases): vestibular migraine? J Neurol. 1999;246(10):883-92.
11. Cass SP, Furman JM, Ankerstjerne K, Balaban C, Yetiser S, Aydogan B. Migraine-related vestibulopathy. Ann Otol Rhinol Laryngol. 1997;106(3):182-9.
12. Lempert T, Olesen J, Furman J, Waterston J, Seemungal B, Carey J, et al. Vestibular migraine: diagnostic criteria. J Vestib Res. 2012;22(4):167-72.
13. Headache Classification Committee of the International Headache Society (IHS). The International Classification of Headache Disorders, 3rd edition (beta version). Cephalalgia. 2013;33(9):629-808.
14. Cutrer FM, Baloh RW. Migraine-associated dizziness. Headache. 1992;32(6):300-4.
15. Kayan A, Hood JD. Neuro-otological manifestations of migraine. Brain. 1984;107(Pt 4): 1123-42.
16. Frohman EM, Kramer PD, Dewey RB, Kramer L, Frohman TC. Benign paroxysmal positioning vertigo in multiple sclerosis: diagnosis, pathophysiology and therapeutic techniques. Mult Scler. 2003;9(3):250-5.
17. Serra A, Chisari CG, Matta M. Eye movement abnormalities in multiple sclerosis: pathogenesis, modeling, and treatment. Front Neurol. 2018;9:31.
18. Kim HA, Lee H. Recent advances in understanding audiovestibular loss of a vascular cause. J Stroke. 2017;19(1):61-6.
19. Pavlou M, Lingeswaran A, Davies RA, Gresty MA, Bronstein AM. Simulator based rehabilitation in refractory dizziness. J Neurol. 2004;251(8):983-95.
20. Strupp M, Brandt T. Central Vertigo. Otorhinolaryngol Clin Int J. 2012;4(2):71-6.
21. Persad AR, Khormi YH, van Landeghem F, Chow MM. Unusual case of hemangioblastoma of the cerebellopontine angle. Surg Neurol Int. 2017;8:264.

11 CHAPTER

Traumatic Vertigo, Vertigo Syndromes, and Psychogenic Vertigo

Natuva Sai S Kumar, Mariappan V, Ganesh Vallampalli, Mugundhan K

ABSTRACT

The illusion of movement of self with environment or movement of the environment with them is vertigo, which can be due to either central or peripheral cause. In this chapter, the author reveals about the various features of traumatic vertigo, vertigo syndromes, and psychogenic dizziness.

INTRODUCTION

Vertigo and imbalance are the common symptoms following head and neck trauma.[1] The incidence ranges from 24 to 83%. Early post-traumatic and delayed post-traumatic are the two types of traumatic vertigo. Early post-traumatic peripheral vertigo includes benign paroxysmal positional vertigo, labyrinthine concussion, and perilymphatic fistula. Delayed post-traumatic vertigo, which occurs 3 weeks to 3 months after trauma, includes Ménière's disease and cervicogenic vertigo.

Benign paroxysmal positional vertigo (BPPV) is diagnosed by sudden onset of vertigo associated with nystagmus, ataxia, and nausea or vomiting on assuming a particular posture. In BPPV, free-floating calcium crystals residing in the canal portion of the semicircular canal (SCC) cause vertigo by exerting a force of heavier otolith debris leading to abnormal fluid endolymph displacement depending upon head position (refer Chapter 8).[2]

Ménière's disease is characterized by sudden, episodic attacks of vertigo associated with fullness of the ear, tinnitus, and unilateral fluctuating hearing loss. The main mechanism is the disruption of the endolymphatic duct secondary to a temporal bone fracture. Displaced epithelia of the sensory end-organs and other cellular elements including the otoconia of the saccule and utricle could result from the shock of trauma.

Post-traumatic central vertigo is caused by vascular diseases of the brainstem, cerebellar infarction, intracranial hemorrhage, and vertebrobasilar insufficiency. They can be caused by a direct concussion of these structures or secondary due to ischemia caused by a traumatic dissection of the vertebral artery.

VESTIBULAR SYNDROMES

Ramsay Hunt Syndrome

The second most common cause of facial palsy following Bell's palsy. It is defined as inflammation of the geniculate ganglion caused by latent Varicella zoster virus resulting in lower motor neuron facial palsy, and vesicular rash of the external ear canal, auricle, and oral cavity. Due to the close proximity of the vestibulocochlear nerve with the geniculate ganglion within the bony facial canal, involvement of the eighth cranial nerve is common resulting in tinnitus, hard of hearing, and vertiginous symptoms.

Unlike Bells' palsy, recovery from facial weakness is <50%. The presence of complete paralysis, age over 50 years, and absent nerve excitability within 1 week of onset resulted in poor recovery. Eyelid synkinesis and perioral synkinesis developed in 60–70% of patients with complete facial palsy, whereas synkinesis of mouth and eye occurred in 10–15% in incomplete palsy.

Ramsay hunt syndrome is a self-limiting illness without any mortality, primary morbidity results from facial weakness. Zoster sine herpete is defined as peripheral facial palsy without ear or mouth rash.

Labyrinthine Concussion

It is defined as sensorineural hearing loss, dizziness, tinnitus, and nystagmus due to injury to the membranous labyrinth following head trauma. Acceleration and deceleration forces generated by head trauma are transmitted to the inner ear producing pulsatile waves resulting in displacement of the basilar membrane, injury to the organ of corti, damage to inner hair cells, and rupture of portions of the membranous labyrinth.

Clinical features include deafness, tinnitus, nystagmus, features of BPPV often accompanied by concussion symptoms and psychotic symptoms. Vestibular symptoms usually resolve within 1 year, if hearing and vertigo persist perilymph fistula should be considered.

A labyrinthine concussion is a clinical diagnosis. Presence of significant craniofacial trauma, trauma to the ear, hearing loss, sudden onset of dizziness after flight, and positive fistula test, one should think of labyrinthine concussion and order for cranial radiography. Complications include anterograde amnesia, frequent headaches, insomnia, photophobia, and concentrating difficulty.

Perilymphatic Fistula

Leakage of perilymph into the middle ear through the oval or round windows, which usually occurs as a complication of stapedectomy or ear surgery, when stapes are dislocated in older days. In the modern era, the etiology proposed was sudden pressure changes in the middle ear due to barotrauma from flying, forceful Valsalva, acoustic trauma, and projectile vomiting. Spontaneous perilymphatic fistula is attributable to a traumatic event which the patient would have forgotten. Intermittent vertigo, fluctuating sensorineural hearing loss, tinnitus, dizziness, and motion intolerance are the most common presenting symptoms.

The volume of perilymph is estimated to be 75 μL, so confirming a leak usually entails visualizing a tiny quantity of fluid. The most commonly employed chemical test to distinguish perilymph from other fluids has been β-transferrin, which is present in perilymph and cerebrospinal fluid, but absent in plasma.

Superior Semicircular Canal Dehiscence

Normally, sound waves enter the fluid-filled inner ear through an oval window and exit via the round window. A deficit of bone overlying the SCC results in a third mobile window effect, leading to an area of increased compliance and movement of endolymph within the canal due to sound and pressure stimulus. Minor, Solomon, and Zee proposed superior semicircular canal dehiscence (SSCD) as a developmental abnormality involving the temporal bone overlying the superior superior semicircular canal (SCC) is unusually thin or absent. Disruption of this thin layer leads to various signs and symptoms **(Fig. 1)**.

Clinical features involve both vestibular and auditory symptoms. Vestibular symptoms include chronic episodic dizziness, pulsatile oscillopsia, vertigo, and nystagmus induced by loud sound (Tullio phenomenon), and vertigo and nystagmus induced by pressure (Hennebert sign). Auditory symptoms include pulsatile tinnitus, mixed hearing loss, and hearing own voice too loudly in the affected ear (autophony). High-resolution computed tomography of the temporal bone and vestibular-evoked myogenic potential are useful in the diagnosis of SSCD.

Cogan's Syndrome

Disorders of young adults in their second and third decade of uncertain etiology are probably associated with large- and medium-sized vessel vasculitis. Hearing loss occurs in two-thirds of patients with progression over a period of 1–3 months.

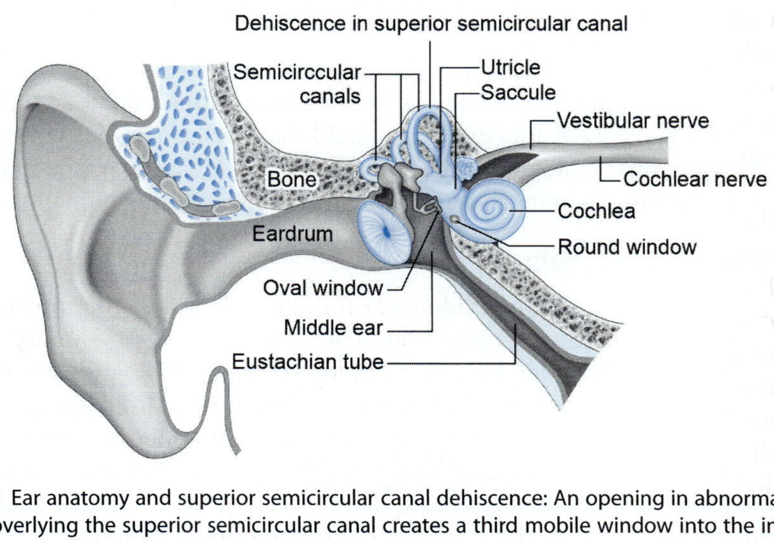

FIG. 1: Ear anatomy and superior semicircular canal dehiscence: An opening in abnormally thin bone overlying the superior semicircular canal creates a third mobile window into the inner ear (in addition to the oval and round windows).

Vertigo, a sensation of fullness in the ear, and vague unsteadiness are other otological manifestations.

Systemic manifestations of Cogan's syndrome include interstitial keratitis, scleritis, episcleritis, aortic insufficiency, fever, generalized body pain, skin rashes, abdominal pain, congestive heart failure, splenomegaly, lymphadenopathy, and hypertension.

Pathogenesis includes humoral and cell-mediated immune response. Antibody response following a viral infection cross-reacts with similar proteins in the eye, inner ear, and other organs due to molecular mimicry. Lymphocyte transformation reaction occurs when patients' lymphocyte is exposed to corneal antigen and inner ear antigen resulting in cell-mediated immunity.

Drug-induced Vertigo

Drugs are also the etiology of vertigo in patients with underlying hepatic and renal compromise. Vestibular ototoxicity affects the balance organs or the vestibular branch of the vestibulocochlear nerve, which can be temporary or permanent. No drug is known to cause Ménière's disease, benign paroxysmal positional vertigo, or any other vestibular disorder causing fluctuating function.

Aspirin, quinine, and loop diuretics produce hearing loss and tinnitus at high doses, which disappear after drug withdrawal. All aminoglycoside antibiotic causes ototoxicity. Some of them cause hearing loss while others cause vestibular loss. A higher risk of ototoxicity occurs in persons receiving dual ototoxic drugs, the presence of decreased kidney function, or has a genetic susceptibility to aminoglycosides. The risk of ototoxicity also increases with an increasing amount of the drug that enters the bloodstream, the longer the drug is in the body, and the duration of time the drug is taken. Aminoglycoside antibiotics can enter the inner ear in all forms, such as intravenous, topical, and inhalational, and cause damage. Antineoplastic drugs causing ototoxicity include cisplatin and carboplatin.

Pathophysiology includes damage to the hair cells and the vestibulocochlear nerve in the inner ear. When "hairs" are normally bent with sound vibrations or movement, they send electrical signals to the brain about hearing or balance function. In ototoxicity, these hairs can be damaged to the point that they no longer stand up, thus reducing the auditory and/or balance signals sent to the brain.

Vestibulotoxicity symptoms range from mild imbalance to total incapacitation. Symptoms depend upon the degree of damage, rapidity, unilateral or bilateral, and duration of the damage that occurred. Slow unilateral damage will not produce any symptoms, but a rapid loss will produce dizziness, vomiting, and nystagmus vestibulotoxicity includes headache, ear fullness, bouncing and blurring of vision,[3] a broad-based gait, difficulty in walking in the dark, lightheadedness, and significant fatigue.

The diagnosis is based upon the patient's history, symptoms, and test results. No specific test is available for a definite diagnosis.[4] Prevention includes avoiding taking multiple types of ototoxic drugs. When using airborne chemicals that are potentially ototoxic, good ventilation should be used.

Vestibular Migraine

Dizziness is one of the most common symptoms affecting 20–30% of the population. Hormonal changes, foods rich in monosodium glutamate, and barometric pressure changes often aggravate both conditions. Dietary changes and medications used in migraine treatment may decrease or prevent the vestibular component of the migraine.

Clinical features include dizziness, recurrent vertigo, tinnitus, photophobia, phonophobia, unsteadiness, cervical muscle spasms, memory disturbance, visuospatial disorientation, and fear. Cortical spreading depression of Leão (a spontaneous spreading of an electrical charge along the cortex) followed by activation of the trigeminovascular system is the key mechanism proposed for migraine. The released neurotransmitters cause vasodilation of scalp blood vessels resulting in pain perception.

Combined auditory and vestibular and function tests are typically used for the evaluation of vestibular migraine.

Episodic Ataxia Type 2

Episodic ataxia type 2 (EA2) is a calcium channelopathy of autosomal-dominant inheritance due to mutations in the *CACNA1A* gene, mapped to chromosome 19p13 resulting in ataxia, vertigo, and nausea typically lasting for minutes to days in duration.

Clinical features are episodic attacks of vertigo, gait, limb ataxia, and nystagmus lasting for minutes to days, with nausea and vomiting without myokymia, triggered by emotional stress, alcohol, caffeine, fever, and heat which respond to acetazolamide therapy. Magnetic resonance imaging of the brain may demonstrate atrophy of the cerebellar vermis with magnetic spectroscopy showing abnormal cerebellar intracellular pH levels and low creatinine. Absent myokymia on electromyography (EMG), and presence of jitter and blocking in single fiber EMG. Molecular genetic testing is used for confirmation of diagnosis.

Variants of *CACNA1A* can cause other disorders, which include familial hemiplegic migraine and spinocerebellar ataxia type 6.

Disembarkment Syndrome

Disorder of imbalance that develops following a sea cruise or aircraft, sleeping on a waterbed, and use of high-speed elevators, which persist for months to years. The most common symptoms are rocking/swaying sensations, dizziness, easy fatigue, poor concentration, and unsteadiness without other vestibular symptoms, such as spinning vertigo, nystagmus, tinnitus, hard of hearing, and double vision.[5] Symptoms are usually aggravated by stress, insomnia, prolonged computer work, and altered barometric pressure.

There is no definite diagnostic test for Mal de debarquement syndrome, it is usually diagnosed by patient history and elimination of other disorders, which may have similar symptoms.

Genetics of Recurrent Vertigo

Mutation involving potassium and calcium channel genes plays a key role in the genesis of recurrent vertigo.

Familial Episodic Ataxias

Most of these ataxias are inherited as autosomal dominant of early onset recurrent attacks of ataxia, dysarthria, and incoordination. Episodic ataxia type 1 is a potassium channelopathy due to a mutation in the *KCNA1* gene on chromosome 12P13 with episodes of vertigo lasting for minutes, diplopia, headache, and dysarthria. Episodic ataxia type 2 is a calcium channelopathy due to a mutation of, the *CACNA1A* gene on chromosome 19p13 with recurrent vertigo lasting for hours to days, ataxia, nystagmus, and migraine.

Episodic ataxia type 3 mapped to chromosome 1q42 with features of vertigo, ataxia, and myokymia. Episodic ataxia type 4 is characterized by vertigo and ataxia, lasting for hours. Episodic ataxia type 5, calcium channelopathy with episodic ataxia and seizures, mapped to chromosome 2q2-23. Episodic ataxia type 6 is characterized by episodic and progressive ataxia, seizures, alternating hemiplegia, and migraine. Episodic ataxia type 7 is characterized by vertigo, weakness, dysarthria, and ataxia lasting for hours to days.

Familial Ménière's Disease

It is inherited as autosomal dominant with incomplete penetrance in around 60% of Ménière's disease. Anticipation is common in familial Ménière's disease, resulting in the early onset of the disease and severe symptoms in successive generations.

Cervical Vertigo

Vertigo or dizziness following a neck injury without hearing impairment. The causes of cervical vertigo are due to vascular compression and altered proprioception.

Vascular Compression

Compression of vertebral arteries, as they pass through the transverse foramen due to cervical spondylotic changes, surgery, or chiropractic manipulation, are the potential causes. Vertebral dissection due to sports injuries and chiropractic manipulation can also lead to cervical vertigo.

Abnormal Sensory Input from Neck Proprioception

Nerves in the neck that sense vibration and movement are proprioceptors. Sensory input from the neck is combined with visual and vestibular information to determine the positions of the head on the neck. Sensory input from the neck also assists in stabilizing vision, which can be elicited by ocular nystagmus from the vibration of the neck.

Diagnosis of cervical vertigo is often uncertain. Other causes of vertigo including central vertigo, inner ear disease, psychogenic vertigo, and medical causes of vertigo should be ruled out before diagnosing cervical vertigo. A magnetic resonance imaging scan of the neck is suggested in all patients with cervical vertigo.

PSYCHOGENIC DIZZINESS AND VERTIGO

Unlocalized vertigo means dizziness that cannot be attributed to an anatomic lesion in a specific place. Anxiety and panic disorder are the most common sources of psychogenic dizziness. Panic disorders are characterized by a sudden inexplicable feeling of terror. People with panic disorders also have vestibular disorders. Psychogenic dizziness responds to benzodiazepine and selective serotonin reuptake inhibitors. About 50% of all dizzy patients have a "functional" source of complaints.

In elderly patients, dizziness without localizing signs are often designated as "presbyastasis," a term synonymous with disequilibrium of aging, which is assigned to persons above the age of 65 years in whom no specific cause of dizziness is identified. Gait disorders should be considered seriously in the elderly. Mechanism of presbyastasis includes progressive degeneration of neural and sensory cells including reduction in hair cell and nerve fiber numbers. Centrally, cerebellar Purkinje cells gradually reduce over life. Neuronal fiber loss also occurs in the extrapyramidal system, the part of the brain that is responsible for movement disorders.

Certain concepts introduced in this chapter have been discussed in Chapter 9 in detail.

CONCLUSION

Post-traumatic vertigo and vertiginous syndromes can result in chronic disabling symptoms resulting in significant morbidity. Most of these syndromes are diagnosed clinically. Before diagnosing psychogenic dizziness, other causes of vertigo should be ruled out.

REFERENCES

1. Griffiths MV. The incidence of auditory and vestibular concussion following minor head injury. J Laryngol Otol. 1979;93(3):253-65.
2. Taneja MK, Vivek T, Himanshu V. Particle repositioning maneuver. Indian J Otol. 2007;13:3-7.
3. Herdman SJ, Tusa RJ, Blatt P, Suzuki A, Venuto PJ, Roberts D. Computerized dynamic visual acuity test in the assessment of vestibular deficits. Am J Otol. 1998;19(6):790-6.
4. Ba'ra'ny R. Nobel Lectures, Physiology or Medicine 1901-1921. Amsterdam: Elsevier Publishing Company; 1967.
5. Grossman GE, Leigh RJ, Abel LA, Lanska DJ, Thurston SE. Frequency and velocity of rotational head perturbations during locomotion. Exp Brain Res. 1988;70(3):470-6.

12 CHAPTER

Approach to Vertigo in Children

Ranjith Kumar Manokaran, Deepti Ashok Kewalramani

ABSTRACT

Vertigo and dizziness in children are challenging clinical symptoms due to their broad differential diagnosis and the child's limited ability to articulate experiences. This chapter outlines a structured approach to evaluating pediatric vertigo, emphasizing the importance of distinguishing true vertigo from pseudovertigo. A thorough history, clinical examination, and appropriate investigations are essential to identify potentially life-threatening conditions such as central nervous system infections, tumors, or cardiovascular disorders. Common benign etiologies like vestibular migraine, benign paroxysmal vertigo of childhood, and postinfectious cerebellar ataxia are also discussed. Practical diagnostic tools such as home video recordings and vestibular maneuvers are highlighted, alongside guidance for neuroimaging and electroencephalography when warranted. Treatment strategies are cause-specific, and management may involve pharmacological, physical, or behavioral interventions.

INTRODUCTION

Giddiness or dizziness is a term not clearly defined which can comprise a variety of conditions, such as light-headedness, ataxia, anxiety, intoxication, hyperventilation, visual disturbance, weakness, depression, and true vertigo. Since the symptoms are vague, it is important to identify benign conditions from potentially serious conditions. It is very difficult for the child to describe the exact quality of the symptoms but can clearly tell the timing and triggers.

DEFINITION

Dizziness/giddiness can be defined as a disturbed sense of relationship to space.[1] Vertigo is an acute symptom that may cause severe alterations in postural control and equilibrium that can be incapacitating to the patient.

CATEGORIZATION

When a child presents with symptoms of apparent vertigo it is important to first differentiate true from pseudovertigo.

- *True vertigo*: It refers to the perception that the patient is rotating relative to the environment (subjective vertigo) or that the environment is rotating relative to the patient (objective vertigo).[2] It results from a disturbance somewhere in the vestibular system, which has both peripheral and central nervous system components.

- *Pseudovertigo*: It describes complaints of dizziness without any rotary component. Common causes include orthostatic hypotension, presyncope, and hyperventilation.

Vertigo and dizziness are dynamic manifestations, which can evolve over time and can represent a sign of complex and/or serious diseases. When approaching a child affected by vertigo, a comprehensive evaluation is crucial to detect the disorder underlying the symptoms and reduce parental anxiety. Home videos recorded by parents can guide the clinician in the diagnostic process since children frequently are unable to explain their experiences.

The most frequent etiologies in all age groups were vestibular migraine (VM) and other variants such as benign paroxysmal vertigo of childhood (BPVC) (recently renamed "recurrent vertigo of childhood"). According to the International Classification of Headache Disorders, BPVC is characterized by recurrent attacks of vertigo resolving spontaneously after minutes to hours.

Migraine is a component present in VM and absent in BPVC. During a child's life, a BPVC diagnosis can switch to VM.

Vestibular neuritis and other vestibular deficits are other common causes.

Postinfectious cerebellar ataxia is recognized as the most frequent cause of acute ataxia in children, and it can also cause symptoms of vertigo or giddiness. Infective involvement of the central nervous system, especially from Herpesviridae and neurotropic bacteria, such as *Borrelia burgdorferi*, can often mimic other neurological conditions. Thus, a prompt diagnosis is a lifesaver in some cases.

Epilepsy, in particular, the vestibular epilepsy subgroup, represents a significant share of neurological causes of vertigo. The manifestations of this type of seizure range from vertigo to tonic-clonic crisis. The electroencephalogram usually demonstrates abnormal epileptiform waves in the temporal lobe.

Central nervous system tumors are the most frequent pediatric solid malignancies and are especially associated with poor prognosis. In subjects suffering from these neoplasms, vertigo, dizziness, and imbalance can be onset signs but also sequelae of surgical or radiation therapy.

Psychogenic vertigo needs to be considered, particularly when dealing with teenagers. Absence from school, relationship issues, and family conflicts can be red flags of possible underlying depression, which requires psychological/psychiatric consultation.

Vertigo associated with cardiovascular disease was found in around 10% of adolescents, representing the third most frequent etiology in older children. Orthostatic vertigo and vasovagal syncope are included among causes of cardiogenic vertigo in most of the series, although in recent years, the rising interest in dysautonomia disorders suggested a correlation between this condition and a failure of the autonomic system. Screening for cardiovascular diseases is highly recommended in consideration of their prognosis and the need for therapy.

Head trauma is a leading cause of accessing pediatric emergency departments and a cause of vertigo, especially in preschool kids. Pathognomonic features such as hemotympanum or Battle sign are suggestive of temporal bone fracture. Imaging is mandatory to delineate the extension of the fracture line and to estimate possible associated damages (i.e., perilymphatic fistula or ossicular chain dislocation).

Patients with a history of head trauma are also recognized to be more prone to develop vestibular disorders, such as BPPV.

Among infrequent causes of vertigo and dizziness, motion sickness accounts for 3.6% of overall diagnoses, alone or as an accompanying manifestation. The cause of this condition is related to a discrepancy between vestibular and ocular signals, and it is usually triggered by car travel or other motion stimuli.

Ophthalmic disorders are also mentioned as possible causes. In this review, their cumulative prevalence is around 1.5%, and it includes a variety of conditions, such as refractive problems or oculomotor dysfunction. Particularly in recent years, the occurrence of vertigo and dizziness in relationship with ophthalmic disorders can be associated with the large use of smartphones among younger individuals, which involves a very demanding visual effort. Orthoptic training and/or correction of the refractive deficit with glasses are easy treatments to perform and, in these cases, lead to a resolution of symptoms.

GENERAL APPROACH

The timing of the symptom, the triggers that provoke the symptom, and a targeted examination (TiTrATE) give a clue to the etiology of giddiness. The common causes of vertigo/dizziness in children and adolescents are listed in **Table 1**.

APPROACH TO PEDIATRIC VERTIGO

History

History should be focused on distinguishing vertigo from pseudovertigo. Though it is difficult for the child to describe, a history of ataxia, vomiting, irritability, desire to lay still, or eye twitching (nystagmus) may indicate true vertigo. History of fever, middle ear infection, altered mental status, toxin exposure, ataxia, hearing loss, vomiting, recent URI, otitis media, recurrence, and recurrent headaches in a family should be asked.

Physical Examination

Findings from the physical examination—including a cardiac and neurologic assessment, with attention to the head, eye, ear, nose, and throat examination—are usually normal in patients presenting with dizziness.

Ear Examination

- Vesicles on the auricle or in the auditory canal (Ramsay Hunt syndrome).
- Tympanic membrane erythema, bulging, or decreased mobility in association with middle ear effusion (otitis media).

TABLE 1: Causes of dizziness in children and adolescents.

	True vertigo	Pseudovertigo
Life-threatening	• CNS infection • Head trauma • Middle ear trauma • Poisoning or adverse medication effect • Stroke • Brain tumor	• Arrhythmia • Heat illness • Hypoglycemia • Poisoning or adverse medication effect
Common	• Benign paroxysmal vertigo of childhood • Labyrinthitis (vestibular neuritis) • Migraine • Motion sickness • Otitis media	• Anemia • Anxiety • Depression • Hyperventilation • Orthostatic hypotension • Pregnancy • Presyncope
Others	• Benign paroxysmal positional vertigo • Cholesteatoma • Congenital defects • Mastoiditis • Ménière's disease • Multiple sclerosis • Perilymph fistula • Ramsay Hunt syndrome • Seizure	Pseudovertigo

- Hemotympanum, otorrhea, tympanic membrane perforation, and/or disruption of the ossicles (temporal bone fracture and/or middle ear injury).
- Swelling, erythema, and tenderness of the mastoid (mastoiditis).
- Vertigo and nystagmus following a loud noise (Tullio phenomenon) or with pneumatic otoscopy of an intact tympanic membrane (perilymphatic fistula).
- Hearing loss (otitis media, mastoiditis, middle ear trauma, and labyrinthitis).

Neurologic Examination

Children with central nervous system infection can have altered sensorium and features of increased intracranial pressure. Meticulous neurologic examination is needed because the presence of a central lesion can be suggested by the presence of additional neurologic abnormalities. A search should be made for cranial nerve abnormalities, motor or sensory changes, dysmetria, or abnormal reflexes. Unilateral peripheral vestibular disorders (e.g., otitis media, benign paroxysmal vertigo) generally cause patients to lean or fall toward the side of the lesion. Children may be uncomfortable and reluctant to move because of their vertigo, but they are still able to walk. Romberg testing will cause the patients to fall or tilt to one side. Patients with an acute cerebellar lesion (e.g., posterior fossa tumor) are often unable to walk without falling. The direction of tilting or falling with Romberg testing may vary.

Provocative Vestibular Testing

- Tests for benign positional vertigo Dix–Hallpike maneuver **(Figs. 1A and B)**.
- Tests of static vestibular imbalance (e.g., skew deviation, ocular tilt reaction, tilt of the subjective visual vertical).
- Tests of dynamic vestibular imbalance (e.g., head thrust test, head shaking visual acuity, and head shaking nystagmus).

Radiology

Neuroimaging is indicated for patients with a history of trauma [computed tomography (CT)] of the head with temporal bone windows or patients with evidence of central vestibular abnormalities, altered mental status, or associated focal neurologic findings [magnetic resonance imaging (MRI) of the brain or head CT]. Once increased intracranial pressure is excluded by physical examination or neuroimaging, lumbar puncture should be performed in patients with suspected meningitis, encephalitis, or multiple sclerosis. In patients with suspicion of seizures, an electroencephalogram should be arranged.

Prolonged or incapacitating vertigo can necessitate other specialized vestibular testing (e.g., electronystagmography, rotary chair testing, posturography, and audiometry). The clinical approach to pseudovertigo and vertigo has been given in **Flowcharts 1 and 2**.

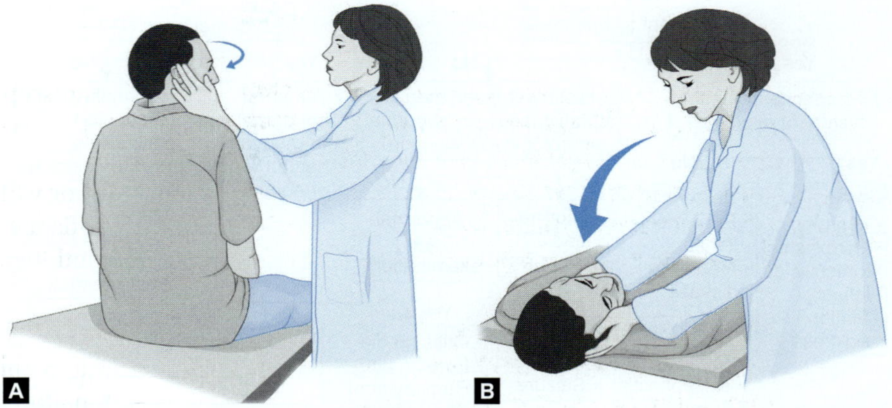

FIGS. 1A AND B: Dix–Hallpike maneuver (used to diagnose benign paroxysmal positional vertigo). This test consists of a series of two maneuvers: (A) With the patient sitting on the examination table, facing forward, eyes open, the physician turns the patient's head 45° to the right and (B) The physician supports the patient's head as the patient lies back quickly from a sitting to supine position, ending with the head hanging 20° off the end of the examination table. The patient remains in this position for 30 seconds. Then the patient returns to the upright position and is observed for 30 seconds. Next, the maneuver is repeated with the patient's head turned to the left. A positive test is indicated if any of these maneuvers trigger vertigo with or without nystagmus.

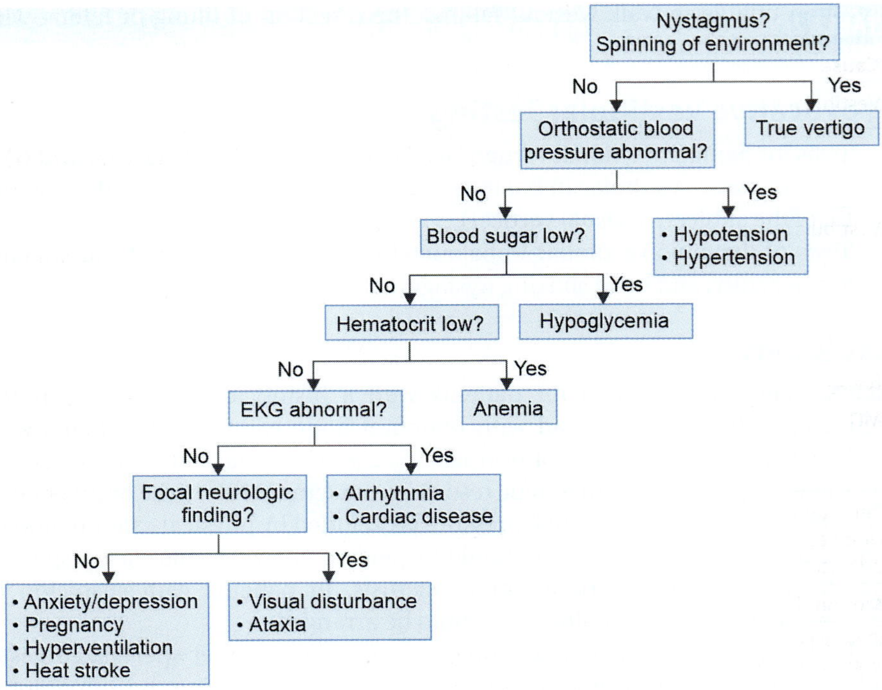

FLOWCHART 1: Approach to pseudovertigo.

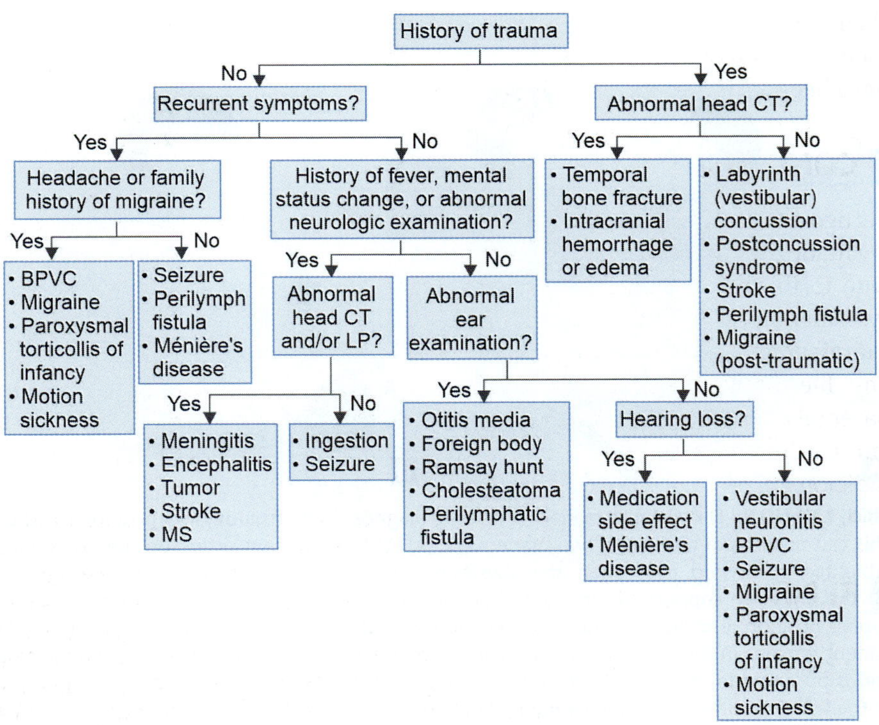

FLOWCHART 2: Approach to the child with true vertigo.

TABLE 2: Various treatment options for vertigo in children.

Cause	Treatment options
Vestibular migraine and recurrent vertigo of childhood	• A prophylaxis is indicated when attacks are more than three per month or if symptoms are severe • Drugs tried—betahistine, flunarizine, topiramate, magnesium, and propranolol
Vestibular neuronitis	• Anti-nausea and antiemesis drugs are available therapeutic options • Dimenhydrinate (1–2 mg/kg) is one of the more viable alternatives, although a short-term usage (3 days maximum) is suggested
BPPV	Epley's maneuver
MD	Several drugs could be used in pediatric patients with MD, e.g., isosorbide dinitrate, dimenhydrinate, diuretics, hydrocortisone, and flunarizine
Persistent postural-perceptual dizziness in children and adolescents	CBT or biofeedback therapy, physical therapy, and SSRI or SNRI have been tried
Motion sickness	Promethazine prophylaxis

(BPPV: benign paroxysmal positional vertigo; CBT: cognitive behavioral therapy; MD: Ménière's disease; SNRI: serotonin noradrenaline reuptake inhibitor; SSRI: selective serotonin reuptake inhibitor)

Treatment of Vertigo in Children

Treatment of vertigo is dependent on the cause of vertigo. Management should be focused based on the etiology and amelioration of symptoms. Specific treatments have been summarized in **Table 2**.

CONCLUSION

Vertigo and dizziness in children are multifactorial symptoms that require careful evaluation to differentiate between benign and serious underlying conditions. Due to the child's developmental limitations in expressing their symptoms, a systematic and vigilant approach involving detailed history, targeted physical examination, and appropriate investigations is vital. Early recognition of treatable and life-threatening causes can significantly improve outcomes and reduce parental anxiety. Clinicians should maintain a high index of suspicion for central and cardiovascular causes when red flags are present and use diagnostic tools judiciously. Ultimately, a tailored, etiology-based management plan ensures optimal care and supports the child's functional recovery and quality of life.

REFERENCES

1. Dizziness. In: Dorland (Ed). Dorland's Medical Dictionary, 29th edition. Philadelphia: WB Saunders; 2000. p. 538.
2. Teach SJ. Dizziness. In: Teach SJ (Ed). Textbook of Pediatric Emergency Medicine, 6th edition. Fleisher GR, Ludwig SL, Henretig FM (Eds). Philadelphia: Lippincott Williams & Wilkins; 2010. p. 226.

13 CHAPTER Medical Therapeutics

Prabash PR, Prabaharan C, Daniel Sweetson A

ABSTRACT

Vertigo is a "symptom" and hence the treatment depends on the etiology of the vertigo. A thorough understanding of vestibular physiology is important for the management of vertigo, and particularly since the clinical picture of a patient with vestibular disorders is continuously evolving. Acute episodes of vertigo are managed with vestibular suppressants and antiemetics. Vestibular suppressants are used only for a shorter duration as prolonged use affects the natural compensatory mechanism.[1,2] Efforts should be made to find the etiology, disease-specific treatment for the causative factor of the vertigo can yield good results. Vestibular rehabilitation therapy (VRT) takes advantage of the innate plasticity of the balance system and speeds up the natural compensation process.

INTRODUCTION

Vertigo, often perceived as a spinning sensation or imbalance, is a symptom with diverse etiologies spanning peripheral and central nervous system disorders. Effective management hinges on a thorough understanding of vestibular physiology and accurate diagnosis of the underlying cause. Treatment strategies range from pharmacological suppression of acute vestibular symptoms to vestibular rehabilitation and disease-specific interventions. A variety of agents—antihistamines, benzodiazepines, anticholinergics, calcium channel blockers, and vestibular stimulants—are employed based on the clinical context. This chapter presents a structured overview of the current therapeutic modalities in vertigo management, emphasizing rational drug use, individualized treatment plans, and emerging interventions across specific vestibular disorders.

TREATMENT OF VERTIGO

Vertigo is a "symptom" and hence the treatment depends on the etiology of the vertigo. A thorough understanding of vestibular physiology is crucial for managing vertigo, especially since the clinical picture of a patient with vestibular disorders is constantly evolving. Vertigo is a multifaceted problem and the management needs a holistic approach.

- *Pharmacotherapy*: It is divided into suppressants for the acute vestibular symptoms and stimulants for the disease-specific treatment of the causative factor of vertigo, as well as enhancing the vestibular compensation process.
- Vestibular rehabilitation therapy (VRT).
- *Adjunctive therapy*: This includes cognitive behavioral therapy, relaxation techniques, breathing exercises, environmental modifications, and safety measures.

In the acute stages, medications are useful in controlling symptoms that last for a few hours to days and are especially useful in relieving autonomic features, such as nausea and vomiting. Acute episodes of vertigo are managed with vestibular suppressants and antiemetics. Vestibular suppressants are used only for a shorter duration as prolonged use affects the natural compensatory mechanism.[1,2]

The medications that are commonly used in the treatment of vertigo are classified into the following groups:

- *Vestibular suppressants*:
  - Antihistamines
  - Benzodiazepines (BZDs)
  - Anticholinergics
  - Calcium channel blockers
  - Antiemetics
- *Vestibular stimulants*: Histamine analogs

VESTIBULAR SUPPRESSANTS

Antihistamines

The mechanism of action of antihistamines in the treatment of vertigo is both by its antihistaminic action and by its anticholinergic activity. The antihistaminic drugs are effective even if given after symptoms have already appeared, unlike pure anticholinergics. All the antihistamines used in the treatment of vertigo cause sedation and due to its potential anticholinergic effect, meclizine must be administered with caution in patients with asthma, glaucoma, or prostate hypertrophy. The commonly used antihistamines are given in **Table 1**.[3]

Benzodiazepines

Benzodiazepines are the next common group of drugs used in the treatment of vertigo. The mechanism of action of benzodiazepine in vertigo is by g-aminobutyric acid (GABA)-mediated vestibular suppression. BZD enhances

TABLE 1: Antihistamine drugs.

Drugs	Dose	Route of administration	Dosing interval	Sedation	Antiemesis
Meclizine	15–50 mg	Oral	4–6 hours	Moderate	Mild
Dimenhydrinate	25–100 mg	Oral, IM, IV	4–8 hours	Moderate	Mild
Promethazine	12.5–25 mg	Oral, IM, rectal	4–12 hours	High	Moderate

(IM: intramuscular; IV: intravenous)

TABLE 2: Benzodiazepines.

Drugs	Dose	Dosing interval	Route	Common adverse effects
Diazepam	5–10 mg	4–6 hourly	Oral, IM, IV	Respiratory depression, sedation, addictive
Lorazepam	0.5–2 mg	6–8 hourly	Oral, IM, IV	Respiratory depression, sedation, addictive
Clonazepam	0.25–0.5 mg	8–12 hourly	Oral	Sedation, addictive

(IM: intramuscular; IV: intravenous)

inhibitory GABA which suppresses the vestibular nuclei and relieves the vertigo symptoms. Although three BZD receptors (Ω1, Ω2, and Ω3) are present in the body, Ω1 agonist is useful in the treatment of vertigo. Diazepam, lorazepam, and clonazepam are the most commonly used BZD. Alprazolam is not used due to its strong withdrawal syndrome. The usefulness of zolpidem (Ω1 agonist) in the treatment of vertigo needs to be studied.[3] The commonly used BZDs are given in **Table 2**.

Anticholinergics

The mechanism of action of anticholinergic drugs is mediated through muscarinic receptors which increases motion tolerance and relieves the symptoms of vertigo. The drugs should have a central anticholinergic effect, i.e., they should cross the blood-brain barrier to relieve the symptoms of vertigo. It also affects compensation, resulting in a reversible overcompensation if administered after attaining central compensation. Scopolamine is the most common anticholinergic agent used in the treatment of vertigo. The dose is 0.5 mg transdermal patch every 3 days. Pure anticholinergics are ineffective if given after symptoms have already appeared, unlike antihistamines. The main side effects of anticholinergics are dry mouth, dilated pupils, and sedation. They should be cautiously used in glaucoma, tachyarrhythmias, and prostate enlargement. Other anticholinergics like glycopyrrolate and zamifenacin need more research for community use.

Calcium Channel Blockers

The calcium channel blockers (CCBs) act both peripherally and centrally. The peripheral action is predominantly by calcium channel blockade whereas the central action is by a combination of calcium channel blockade, anticholinergic, and antihistaminic properties of the drugs.[4-7] Flunarizine and cinnarizine are the common calcium channel blockers used in the treatment of vertigo. They are useful in conditions where migraine and vertigo coexist as they are used in the treatment of migraine also.

The fixed combination of cinnarizine 20 mg with dimenhydrinate 40 mg has recently been used in the treatment of acute vertigo. Its efficacy far exceeded that of equally dosed other drugs used in the treatment of vertigo, leading to higher responder rates. The tolerability and adverse effect profile are similar to other agents. Some of the CCBs used in the treatment of vertigo are given in **Table 3**.[3]

TABLE 3: Calcium channel blockers.				
Drugs	**Dose**	**Route**	**Dosing interval**	**Common adverse effects**
Cinnarizine	25 mg	Oral	8 hourly	Sedation and headache
Flunarizine	10 mg	Oral	At bedtime	Sedation and headache
Nimodipine	30 mg	Oral	12 hourly	Headache and flushing
Verapamil	120 mg	Oral	At bedtime	Constipation

TABLE 4: Antiemetic drugs.		
Drugs	**Dose**	**Common adverse effects**
Antihistamines		
Meclizine	12.5–25 mg QID 4–6 hourly PO	Sedation, use with caution in glaucoma and prostate enlargement
5-HT antagonist		
Granisetron	1 mg PO/1 mg IV	Headache
Ondansetron	• 4–8 mg PO 8 mg sublingual • 4–16 mg IV	Headache, diarrhea, and fever
Palonosetron	0.25 mg IV	Headache and constipation
Metoclopramide	10 mg PO TID or 10 mg IM	Restlessness, drowsiness, and extrapyramidal effects
Phenothiazines		
Prochlorperazine	5–10 mg IM or PO 6–8 hourly/25 rectal QID 12 hourly	Sedation and extrapyramidal effects
Promethazine	25 mg PO QID 6–8 hours or 25 mg rectal QID 12 hours or 12.5 mg IM QID 6–8 hours	Sedation and extrapyramidal effects
Thiethylperazine	10 mg PO, up to TID or 10 mg IM, up to TID	Sedation and extrapyramidal effects

(QID: four times a day; PO: per os; TID: thrice a day; IM: intramuscular; IV: intravenous)

Antiemetics

Antiemetics are used to control vomiting and nausea associated with vertigo. Routinely antiemetics are not prescribed separately for vertigo as most of the antihistaminic drugs have antiemetic properties. The choice of antiemetic drug depends on the severity of vomiting, route of administration, and adverse effects. The most commonly used antiemetic is meclizine, which has both antiemetic and antihistaminic properties with minimal side effects. Other second-line drugs like phenothiazines, which have effective antiemetic properties, are not commonly used because of extrapyramidal side effects. The 5-hydroxytryptamine (5-HT) antagonists and drugs that speed gastric emptying such as metoclopramide may also be helpful in managing vomiting. The list of antiemetic drugs is given in **Table 4**.

VESTIBULAR STIMULANTS

Histamine Analogs

Betahistine is a weak H1 and H2 receptor agonist and a moderate H3 antagonist (presynaptic). Betahistine acts peripherally by reducing the asymmetric functioning of the sensory vestibular organs in addition to increasing vestibulocochlear blood flow by antagonizing local H3 receptors. Betahistine acts centrally by enhancing histamine synthesis within tuberomammillary nuclei of the posterior hypothalamus and histamine release within vestibular nuclei through antagonism of H3 autoreceptors. This mechanism, together with the effects of betahistine on alertness regulation through cerebral H1 receptors, facilitates central vestibular compensation.[8-10] The recommended dose is 16–24 mg TDS. Betahistine is contraindicated in people with pheochromocytoma and hepatic dysfunction. People with bronchial asthma and a history of peptic ulcers need to be closely monitored. Betahistine should be used with caution in pregnancy **(Table 5)**.

Other Agents

Various other agents are used in the treatment of vertigo with unknown mechanisms and efficacy. *Ginkgo biloba* is a newer entry in the treatment of vertigo. The mechanism of action is unclear, and it is postulated that by reducing the viscosity of blood, it improves inner ear circulation and thereby reduces vertigo symptoms. Recent studies have shown that *Ginkgo biloba* is as effective as betahistine in the treatment of vertigo.[11,12]

The other agents used in the treatment of vertigo are given in **Table 6**.[3]

TABLE 5: Dose, route, and adverse effects of betahistine hydrochloride.

Drugs	Dose	Route	Dosing interval	Common adverse effects
Betahistine hydrochloride	8, 16, and 24 mg	Oral	For 8 and 16 mg—8 hourly; for 24 mg—12 hourly	Headache, nausea, and dyspepsia

TABLE 6: Other drugs used in vertigo.

Drug	Dosage	Mechanism of action	Common side effects
Ginkgo biloba	120–240 mg/day	Unknown. Reduces the viscosity of blood	Allergy, interaction with blood thinners
Baclofen	10–80 mg/day	Gamma-aminobutyric acid (GABA) agonist	Gastritis, weakness
Amantadine	100 mg OD or BD	Dopamine agonist	Rashes
Piracetam	800 mg BD or TDS	Not known	Tremor, confusion, anxiety, and insomnia

(BD: twice a day; OD: once a day; TDS: thrice a day)

TABLE 7: Agents that need further evaluation.

Drugs	Mechanism of action	Current status
Pentoxifylline	Not known weak tumor necrosis factor inhibitor	Needs further studies
Phenytoin	Sodium channel blocker	Needs further studies
DL-leucine	Restores the symmetry of central vestibular neurons	Needs further studies
3,4-diaminopyridine	Potassium channel blocker used to reduce downbeat nystagmus in vertigo	Needs further studies
Isosorbide	Unknown mechanism? osmotic diuretic	Needs further studies

Agents that Need Further Evaluation

A few agents that are tried in the treatment of vertigo and their possible mechanism of action are given in **Table 7**.

TREATMENT OF SPECIFIC DISORDERS

Benign Paroxysmal Positional Vertigo

Benign paroxysmal positional vertigo (BPPV) arises from canalolithiasis caused by otoconia (calcite crystals) which get dislodged from the utricle and move freely in the semicircular canals. Although physical treatment is the treatment of choice, antiemetics has a role in reducing nausea and vomiting. Antiemetics are given before various physical treatments. Meclizine or prochlorperazine are commonly used drugs that have both antiemetic and antivertiginous properties.[13]

The Epley maneuver used to treat posterior semicircular canal (PSC)-BPPV consists of stepwise 90° rotations of the head toward the unaffected side. The Epley maneuver is performed in five steps, including two from the Dix–Hallpike maneuver, and is described in Chapter 14.

The Semont maneuver is an alternative method for treating PSC-BPPV mainly in patients with back pain who cannot do the Epley maneuver. During this maneuver, the patient makes rapid sweeping movement from the affected to the unaffected side.[13]

Geotropic horizontal semicircular canal (HSC)-BPPV is treated by:

- Log roll exercise in which the patient's head is rotated 270° with sequential 90° turns from the affected ear down position to the prone position.[13]
- The Gufoni maneuver in which the patient lies to the side from a sitting position with the unaffected ear down, head turning toward the floor, and resuming the sitting position with each position maintained for 1–2 minutes.[14]

Apogeotropic HSC-BPPV is also treated by the Gufoni maneuver in which the patient sits upright, looking straight, and then quickly lies down on the affected side. Then the patient remains in this position for 1–2 minutes. Then the head is quickly turned 45° toward the ceiling and held in this same position for 2 minutes, after which the patient slowly resumes the sitting position.[14]

Yacovino maneuver is used for treating anterior canal (AC)-BPPV, which consists of gradual lifting of the overextended head in a head-down position, followed by sitting up.[15]

Vestibular Neuritis

Recent studies have shown that recovery of peripheral vestibular function was significantly improved with methylprednisolone 100 mg/day and tapered to 10 mg/day over 3 weeks. This trend, 1 month after illness was also discerned in a Cochrane review, but no general recommendation for corticosteroid treatment was given because of the insufficient number of studies. If the patients are suffering from severe nausea and retching, vestibular suppressants and antiemetics like prochlorperazine can be administered for the first few days to relieve the symptoms. Prolonged administration is not advised as it delays central compensation. The efficacy of physiotherapy with dynamic exercises for balance regulation and of gaze stabilization for improvement of central vestibulospinal compensation has been proven in many studies.[16,17]

Bilateral Vestibulopathy

The three common causes are ototoxic drugs, bilateral Ménière's disease, and meningitis.[18] They are symptom-free when sitting or lying. Treatment options include:

- Ototoxic drugs such as aminoglycosides, and furosemide should be stopped and avoided.
- Avoid using vestibular suppressants as they worsen the condition by interfering with central compensation.
- Avoid loud noise.
- Vestibular exercises.

MÉNIÈRE'S DISEASE

The acute symptoms of vertigo, nausea, and vomiting can be treated with antihistamines and antiemetics. For mild symptoms oral Meclizine, prochlorperazine, diazepam, and clonazepam are used. For severe attacks, parenteral promethazine and prochlorperazine can be used.

Prophylactic treatment options for reducing the frequency of attacks are:

- Long-term high-dose (48 mg TDS) administration of betahistine[19-21]
- Transtympanic instillation of gentamicin and of steroids.[22-24]

If high-dose treatment with betahistine fails to achieve any improvement, transtympanic gentamicin may be successful. Gentamicin takes effect by causing direct damage to vestibular type I hair cells. Other supportive treatment includes the use of mild diuretics like hydrochlorothiazide and triamterene, carbonic anhydrase inhibitors like acetazolamide, and spironolactone in women with premenstrual flare-ups. In the elderly, diuretics should be used with caution as it can cause hyponatremia. Hence, frequent electrolyte monitoring is needed.

Lifestyle modifications such as avoiding smoking, avoiding caffeine, and a salt-restricted diet may help to reduce the symptoms. The surgical option is preferred if conservative management fails.

VESTIBULAR MIGRAINE

An acute attack of migraine is treated with nonsteroidal anti-inflammatory drugs (NSAIDs), triptans (sumatriptan, naratriptan, eletriptan, zolmitriptan, rizatriptan, etc.), antihistamines, and antiemetics. Sumatriptan and naproxen fixed dose combination is also available. Drugs used in the treatment of migraine prophylaxis are given in **Table 8.**[25]

VESTIBULAR PAROXYSMIA

Vestibular paroxysmia probably arises from neurovascular compression of the seventh cranial nerve in the vicinity of the brainstem due to crosstalk between partly demyelinizedaxons.[26-28] If the patient has more than two attacks per month, low-dose carbamazepine 200–600 mg/day may be used. Phenytoin and valproic acid are alternatives for patients who do not tolerate carbamazepine, but the efficacy of these agents is not studied in trials with larger populations.

TABLE 8: Drugs used in the treatment of migraine.

Drugs	Dosage	Adverse effects
Tricyclics		
Amitriptyline	10–75 mg HS	Drowsiness
Nortriptyline	25–75 mg HS	–
Dosulepin (dothiepin)	25–75 mg HS	–
Beta-blockers		
Propranolol	40–120 mg BD	• Postural symptoms • Contraindicated in asthma
Anticonvulsants		
Sodium valproate	400–600 mg BD	Hematologic/hepatic/fetal abnormalities, weight gain, tremors
Topiramate	25–200 mg per day	Paresthesia, nephrolithiasis, weight loss, and glaucoma
Gabapentin	900–3600 mg QID	Sedation
Others		
Flunarizine	5–15 mg QID	Depression, weight gain, and extrapyramidal features
Methysergide	1–4 mg QID	Drowsiness, cramps, and retroperitoneal fibrosis

(QID: four times a day; BD: twice a day)

CEREBELLAR AND CENTRAL VERTIGO SYNDROMES

Aminopyridines (potassium-channel blockers)[29-32] have become established as a new pharmacological treatment option for the following symptoms of cerebellar diseases:

- Downbeat nystagmus
- Central positional nystagmus
- Episodic ataxia type 2
- Gait disorders in cerebellar ataxia

Either 4-aminopyridine (5 mg/day BD/TDS) or its slow-release form fampridine (10 mg/day OD/BD) is used in various studies to treat cerebellar vertigo syndromes. In addition to aminopyridines and acetazolamide (125–1,000 mg) have been used in the treatment of episodic ataxia type 2. Other causes for central vertigo such as transient ischemic attacks, vertebrobasilar insufficiency, and central demyelination should be treated for their cause.

CONCLUSION

The management of vertigo requires a nuanced understanding of its pathophysiological underpinnings and a diagnosis-driven therapeutic strategy. While pharmacological agents offer symptomatic relief during acute episodes, they must be judiciously used to avoid hindering central compensation. Disease-specific treatments, such as repositioning maneuvers for BPPV, corticosteroids for vestibular neuritis, and betahistine or intratympanic therapies for Ménière's disease, enhance outcomes when appropriately applied. Additionally, non-pharmacological adjuncts, including behavioral therapy and lifestyle modifications, contribute significantly to holistic care.

REFERENCES

1. Yacovino DA, Carrea R, Luis L. Pharmacologic treatment of vestibular disorders. Vestibular Disorders Association. [online] Available from www.vestibular.org [Last accessed April, 2025].
2. Strupp M, Thurtell MJ, Shaikh AG, Brandt T, Zee DS, Leigh RJ. Pharmacotherapy of vestibular and ocular motor disorders, including nystagmus. J Neurol. 2011;258(7):1207-22.
3. Hain TC, Yacovino D. Pharmacologic treatment of persons with dizziness. Neurol Clin. 2005;23(3):831-85.
4. Lee JA, Watson LA, Boothby G. Calcium antagonists in the prevention of motion sickness. Aviat Space Environ Med. 1986;57(1):45-8.
5. Olesen J. Calcium entry blockers in the treatment of vertigo. Ann N Y Acad Sci. 1988;522: 690-7.
6. Tolu E, Mameli O, Caria MA, Melis F. Improvement of vestibular plasticity in the guinea pig with a calcium entry blocker. Acta Otolaryngol (Stockh). 1988;460:72-9.
7. Verspeelt J, De Locht P, Amery WK. Postmarketing study of the use of flunarizine in vestibular vertigo and in migraine. Eur J Clin Pharmacol. 1996;51(1):15-22.
8. Lacour M, Sterkers O. Histamine and betahistine in the treatment of vertigo: Elucidation of mechanisms of action. CNS Drugs. 2001;15(11):853-70.
9. Mira E. Betahistine in the treatment of vertigo. History and clinical implications of recent pharmacological researches. Acta Otorhinolaryngol Ital. 2001;66(Suppl):1-7.
10. Mira E, Guidetti G, Ghilardi PL, Fattori B, Malannino N, Maiolino L, et al. Betahistine dihydrochloride in the treatment of peripheral vestibular vertigo. Eur Arch Otorhinolaryngol. 2003;260(2):73-7.

11. Cesarani A, Meloni F, Alpini D, Barozzi S, Boscani PF, Verderio L, et al. Ginkgo biloba (EGb 761) in the treatment of equilibrium disorders. Adv Ther. 1998;15(5):291-304.
12. Sokolova L, Hoerr R, Mishchenko T. Treatment of vertigo: a randomized, double-blind trial comparing efficacy and safety of Ginkgo biloba extract EGb 761 and betahistine. Int J Otolaryngol. 2014;2014:682439.
13. Jung I, Kim JS. Approach to dizziness in the emergency department. Clin Exp Emerg Med. 2015;2(2):75-88.
14. Gufoni M, Mastrosimone L. Repositioning maneuver in benign paroxysmal vertigo of horizontal semicircular canal. Acta Otorhinolaryngol Ital. 1998;18(6):363-7.
15. Yacovino DA, Hain TC, Gualtieri F. New therapeutic maneuver for anterior canal benign paroxysmal positional vertigo. J Neurol. 2009;256(11):1851-5.
16. Strupp M, Zingler VC, Arbusow V, Niklas D, Maag KP, Dieterich M, et al. Methylprednisolone, valacyclovir, or the combination for vestibular neuritis. N Engl J Med. 2004;351(4):354-61.
17. Fishman JM, Burgess C, Waddell A. Corticosteroids for the treatment of idiopathic acute vestibular dysfunction (vestibular neuritis). Cochrane Database Syst Rev. 2011;5:CD008607.
18. Zingler VC, Cnyrim C, Jahn K, Weintz E, Fernbacher J, Frenzel C, et al. Causative factors and epidemiology of bilateral vestibulopathy in 255 patients. Ann Neurol. 2007;61(6):524-32.
19. Strupp M, Huppert D, Frenzel C, Wagner J, Hahn A, Jahn K, et al. Long-term prophylactic treatment of attacks of vertigo in Meniere's disease—comparison of a high with a low dosage of betahistine in an open trial. Acta Otolaryngol. 2008;128(5):520-4.
20. Lezius F, Adrion C, Mansmann U, Jahn K, Strupp M. High-dosage betahistine dihydrochloride between 288 and 480 mg/day in patients with severe Menière's disease: a case series. Eur Arch Otorhinolaryngol. 2011;268(8):1237-40.
21. Ihler F, Bertlich M, Sharaf K, Strieth S, Strupp M, Canis M. Betahistine exerts a dose-dependent effect on cochlear stria vascularis blood flow in Guinea pigs in vivo. PLoS One. 2012;7(6):e39086.
22. Pullens B, van Benthem PP. Intratympanic gentamicin for Ménière's disease or syndrome. Cochrane Database Syst Rev. 2011;3:CD008234.
23. Garduno-Anaya MA, Couthino De TH, Hinojosa-Gonzalez R, Pane-Pianese C, Rios-Castaneda LC. Dexamethasone inner ear perfusion by intratympanic injection in unilateral Ménière's disease: a two-year prospective, placebo-controlled, double-blind, randomized trial. Otolaryngol Head Neck Surg. 2005;133(2):285-94.
24. Casani AP, Piaggi P, Cerchiai N, Seccia V, Franceschini SS, Dallan I. Intratympanic treatment of intractable unilateral Meniere disease: gentamicin or dexamethasone? A randomized controlled trial. Otolaryngol Head Neck Surg. 2012;146(3):430-7.
25. Lempert T, Olesen J, Furman J, Waterston J, Seemungal B, Carey J, et al. Vestibular migraine: diagnostic criteria—consensus document of the Bárány Society and the International Headache Society. Nervenarzt. 2013;84(4):511-6.
26. Brandt T, Dieterich M. Vestibular paroxysmia: vascular compression of the eighth nerve? Lancet. 1994;343(8900):798-9.
27. Strupp M, von Stuckrad-Barre S, Brandt T, Tonn JC. Teaching neuroimages: compression of the eighth cranial nerve causes vestibular paroxysmia. Neurology. 2013;80(7):e77.
28. Hüfner K, Barresi D, Glaser M, Linn J, Adrion C, Mansmann U, et al. Vestibular paroxysmia: diagnostic features and medical treatment. Neurology. 2008;71(13):1006-14.
29. Strupp M, Schüler O, Krafczyk S, Jahn K, Schautzer F, Büttner U, et al. Treatment of downbeat nystagmus with 3,4-diaminopyridine: a placebo-controlled study. Neurology. 2003;61(2):165-7.
30. Kremmyda O, Zwergal A, la Fougère C, Brandt T, Jahn K, Strupp M. 4-Aminopyridine suppresses positional nystagmus caused by cerebellar vermis lesion. J Neurol. 2013;260(1):321-3.
31. Strupp M, Kalla R, Claassen J, Adrion C, Mansmann U, Klopstock T, et al. A randomized trial of 4-amino- pyridine in EA2 and related familial episodic ataxias. Neurology. 2011;77:269-75.
32. Schniepp R, Wuehr M, Neuhaeusser M, Benecke AK, Adrion C, Brandt T, et al. 4-Aminopyridine and cerebellar gait: a retrospective case series. J Neurol. 2012;259(11):2491-3.

14 CHAPTER

Vestibular Rehabilitation

Deepa Avadhani, Hemanth Kumar Arumugam, Bagath Srinivasan Balaji

ABSTRACT

Vertigo is a common symptom encountered in neurological practice. Vestibular rehabilitation makes use of inherent plasticity of whole balance system to enhance the process of natural eye and head movements to hasten the recovery. It includes physical therapy and canalith repositioning techniques. The three main principles of vestibular rehabilitation include adaptation, substitution, and habituation. This chapter gives some insights into the exercises and repositioning techniques of vestibular rehabilitation. These strategies are complementary to pharmacotherapy in patient recovery. These are useful in peripheral as well as central vestibular disorders.

INTRODUCTION

Vertigo is a common complaint encountered in neurological practice. It is observed that vertigo due to vestibular lesions often has a benign cause, which can be self-limiting or be relieved by the process of compensation by the central nervous system. Neuronal discharges from the brainstem and cerebellum are responsible for the compensation. Sometimes, poor compensation and maladaptive posture can be present even in the absence of ongoing vestibular pathology. Vestibular rehabilitation makes use of the inherent plasticity of the whole balance system to enhance the process of natural movements of the head and eyes to hasten the recovery.[1] The vestibular rehabilitation includes two categories: (1) Physical therapy for vestibular dysfunction, which is also known as vestibular rehabilitation therapy and (2) Canalith repositioning techniques for benign paroxysmal positional vertigo (BPPV).

Indications for vestibular rehabilitation:

- Unilateral or bilateral vestibular hypofunction
- Otolith disorders
- Vestibular neuritis
- Labyrinthitis
- Persistent postural-perceptual dizziness (PPPD)
- Central vestibular disorders

Deciding factors for vestibular rehabilitation:[2]

- Age of the patient
- Site of the lesion
- Severity of the disease
- Etiology

PRINCIPLES OF VESTIBULAR REHABILITATION

Treatment of the patients with acute vestibular neuritis or acute labyrinthitis may include vestibular suppressants and antiemetics, but there is lack of sufficient evidence for the use of medication in patients with chronic vestibular hypofunction. In these chronic cases, the treatment is primarily based on exercises. Low-dose antihistamines for short duration for symptomatic relief may not cause significant harm. A surgical approach or ablative approach has limited applications in patients who have fluctuating vestibular function and recurrent vertigo. In the 1940s, Cawthorne and Cooksey developed the original vestibular exercises and these are designed to reduce the symptoms of motion-induced dizziness. These exercises are standardized and include a progression of only eye movements, movements of the head with open eyes or closed eyes, bending over, sitting and standing, tossing a small ball, climbing a ladder, and walking. The patient's position progresses from lying-down position, to sitting, then standing, and finally, walking. Recently, these exercises have been combined with modern techniques to enhance the recovery.[3]

Vestibular rehabilitation is based on three main principles: (1) Vestibular adaptation, (2) vestibular substitution, and (3) habituation **(Flowchart 1)**:

- *Adaptation:* Instability of the gaze is due to the reduced gain of the vestibular response to head movements. Retinal slip (image motion on the retina during the movements of head) is the best stimulus to increase the gain of vestibular response. It can be induced by vertical or horizontal head movements with visual fixation on a target. The target can be kept either across the room or within an arm's length. Repeated periods of retinal slip lead to vestibular adaptation. There are many ways to enhance the effect of vestibular adaptation. Different amplitudes of retinal slip should be used. Progressive increase in retinal slip errors is more effective. To enhance the magnification and the exposure duration to retinal slip, the subject is asked to view a moving target, the direction of which is opposite to the direction of the head movement. It is noticed that greatest changes in vestibulo-ocular reflex (VOR) gain occur in training frequencies. It is advisable to apply a wide range of frequencies of head movements. It is also important to employ different directions of head movements, as this would give an otolithic input, which can influence the training effects.
- *Substitution:* Substitution by other eye-movement systems can effectively protect the patient from perceiving smeared images during movements and cancel the vestibular deficit. It includes saccade modification and enhancement of pursuit movements. Corrective saccades are a part of adaptive strategy

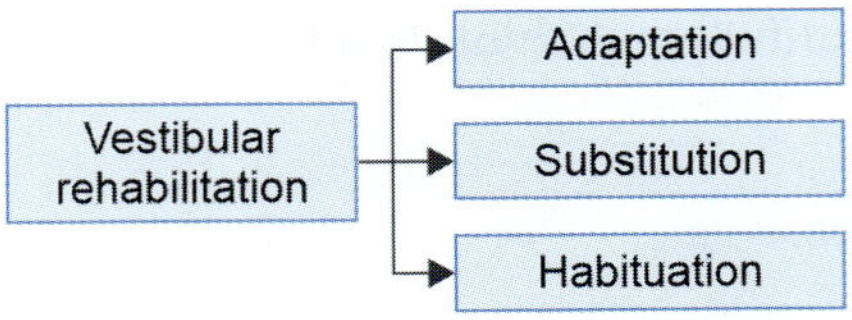

FLOWCHART 1: Principles of vestibular rehabilitation.

to enhance the slow component of VOR. When a patient follows the target, saccade to the target of lesser amplitude (undershoot) is generated, which is of insufficient amplitude, and after that, the eyes drift to the target helping to keep the eye position fixed during head movements. The other saccade is a preprogrammed saccade. During an ipsilesional sudden head rotation away from the target, the saccade will be formed in the direction opposite to the head rotation and back toward the target. By enhancing smooth-pursuit eye movement and deficit of VOR can be substituted. Patients with bilateral vestibular loss use smooth pursuit system to maintain gaze stability.

- *Habituation:* Habituation happens after repeatedly exposing a person to a provocative stimulus, which will result in reduction of symptoms over a period of time. Physiologically, habituation is a result of reduced excitatory postsynaptic potential due to the effect of calcium channel blockers on presynaptic membrane, while adaptation is the result of upregulated expression of genes resulting in tissue remodeling.

EXERCISES FOR VESTIBULAR REHABILITATION

Gaze stabilization exercises (GSEs): They are based on the principles of VOR adaptation and VOR substitution. Vestibular adaptation is the result of the long-term modification in the neuronal firing rate in response to the head movements with the intent of decreasing retinal slip. Clinically, the change in neuronal firing rate leads to normalization of gaze stability, normalization of postural stability, and reduction of symptoms. GSEs based on the concept of vestibular adaptation are known as adaptation exercises. They include movement of the head while keeping the focus on a particular target, which may be moving or stationary. GSEs based on the concept of vestibular substitution are known as substitution exercises and they promote alternate strategies, which substitute for lost vestibular function.[1] The alternate strategies include central preprogramming of eye movements or compensatory saccades. For example, when the active eye-head exercise is performed between the targets, a large amplitude eye movement to the target is made before the head movement to face the target, facilitating the application of preprogrammed eye movements. Adaptation exercises and substitution exercises are performed with head movements in both the horizontal and vertical planes.

The dose of GSEs differs in acute versus chronic cases. The exercises have to be done at least 3 times a day in both the cases. However, the total duration should be at least 12 minutes per day in acute cases and 20 minutes per day in chronic cases.

Habituation refers to the reduction in a behavioral response after repetitive exposure to a stimulus.[1] Habituation exercises are based on particular movements or situations that provoke symptoms. The patient performs repetitions of visual or body movements that result in mild-to-moderate-symptoms. This repetition of provocative movements leads habituation and symptom reduction over time. Recent approach to habituation involves advanced technology utilizing optokinetic stimulation (OKS) and virtual reality (VR) or balance exercises. OKS uses optokinetic discs or videos or moving rooms to provide repetitive motion patterns. VR immerses the patients in a realistic and visually challenging environment. It may involve activities including no immersive gaming also. Stimulus parameters such as direction of stimulus motion, velocity, size, color, and cognitive load may help grade the stimulus intensity in both these approaches. Balance challenges can be added by making the patient engage in the VR or OKS activities while walking, standing, balancing, or weight shifting.

Balance and gait training is an important aspect of vestibular rehabilitation. They optimize the postural control systems. They encompass exercises for center of gravity control, reactive and anticipatory balance control, gait exercises, and multisensory training. Exercises for center of gravity control include shifting of weight in stance and/or changing the base of support (e.g., tandem, Romberg, and single leg stance) to enhance the challenge. Reactive and anticipatory balance exercises include the training of various strategies of balance recovery (e.g., hip, ankle, or stepping strategy) under involuntary and voluntary conditions. Multisensory balance exercises include balancing under different input conditions including altered vestibular (e.g., head movement), visual (e.g., OKS), and somatosensory (e.g., moving surfaces) stimuli. Gait exercises include dynamic conditions like conducting a secondary task (e.g., counting backward) while walking or walking with head turns. Patient-reported balance rating scale may help in the assessment of progress.

Advanced technology may help augment gait and balance training. Different gaming techniques can be fun for the patients. At the same time, they work on both postural control and VOR gain, simultaneously, if the patient is standing. Platform perturbations can be used to increase the postural control in standing. Vibrotactile stimulation gives sensory information through an alternate sensory modality to augment or replace a defective sense. The aim is to provide the patient with information about the position of body in space through a waist belt, which has vibrating sensors. Vibrotactile feedback is used to alert the patient when there is excessive tilt from the predetermined vertical. General conditioning exercises complement the earlier-mentioned exercises and include graduated and customized walking program for endurance.

REPOSITIONING MANEUVERS

Benign paroxysmal positional vertigo can be classified based on the affected canal into three types: (1) Posterior canal BPPV, (2) lateral or horizontal canal BPPV, and (3) anterior canal BPPV. Repositioning maneuvres are mainstay of treatment for BPPV **(Flowchart 2)**.

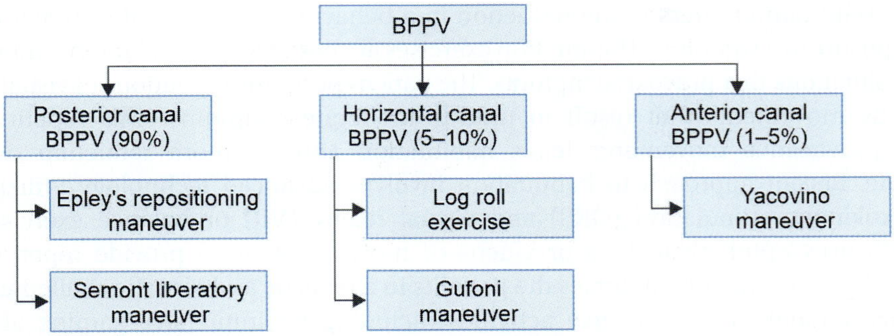

FLOWCHART 2: Classification and repositioning maneuvers of benign paroxysmal positional vertigo (BPPV).

Posterior Canal Benign Paroxysmal Positional Vertigo

Modified Epley's maneuver:[4,5] Using the Dix–Hallpike maneuver, the affected canal is localized first. This technique is for the right-sided inner ear pathology **(Figs. 1A to H)**.

Semont's maneuver:[6] The Semont's maneuver is illustrated in **(Figs. 2A to C)**.

Lateral Canal Benign Paroxysmal Positional Vertigo

Gufoni-Appiani maneuver: This maneuver is used when the patient has geotropic nystagmus on supine roll test and is associated with the presence of otoliths in the posterior arm of the semicircular canal.[7] The individual is seated at the center of the table. The individual quickly lays on the side with the damaged ear down. The individual maintains this position until the disappearance of nystagmus. The doctor turns the individual's head 45° upward and holds it in this position for 2 minutes. Then, the individual slowly returns to the sitting position.

Cupulolith repositioning maneuver: It is done when the patient has apogeotropic nystagmus on supine roll test and is associated with the presence of otoliths in anterior arm of the semicircular canal. With the individual in the supine position, the head is turned 90° toward the affected side. A vibrator (60 Hz) is placed on the posterosuperior aspect of the affected inner ear for 30 seconds and this position is maintained for 2 minutes. The head is turned 90° toward the normal side quickly (upright position) and is held like this for 2 minutes. The head is then quickly turned 90° toward the normal side (position of the affected inner ear facing the ceiling), a vibrator (60 Hz) is placed on the posterosuperior aspect of the affected inner ear for 30 seconds, and this position is maintained for 2 minutes. Then the head is turned 90° toward the normal side (prone) and is held in this position for 2 minutes. The patient sits slowly with head slightly bowed.

Anterior Canal Benign Paroxysmal Positional Vertigo

It is a very rare type of BPPV and is diagnosed by the presence of vertical downbeating nystagmus with or without torsional component. The Yacovino maneuver can be used in this type.[8] The patient is first placed in a sitting position

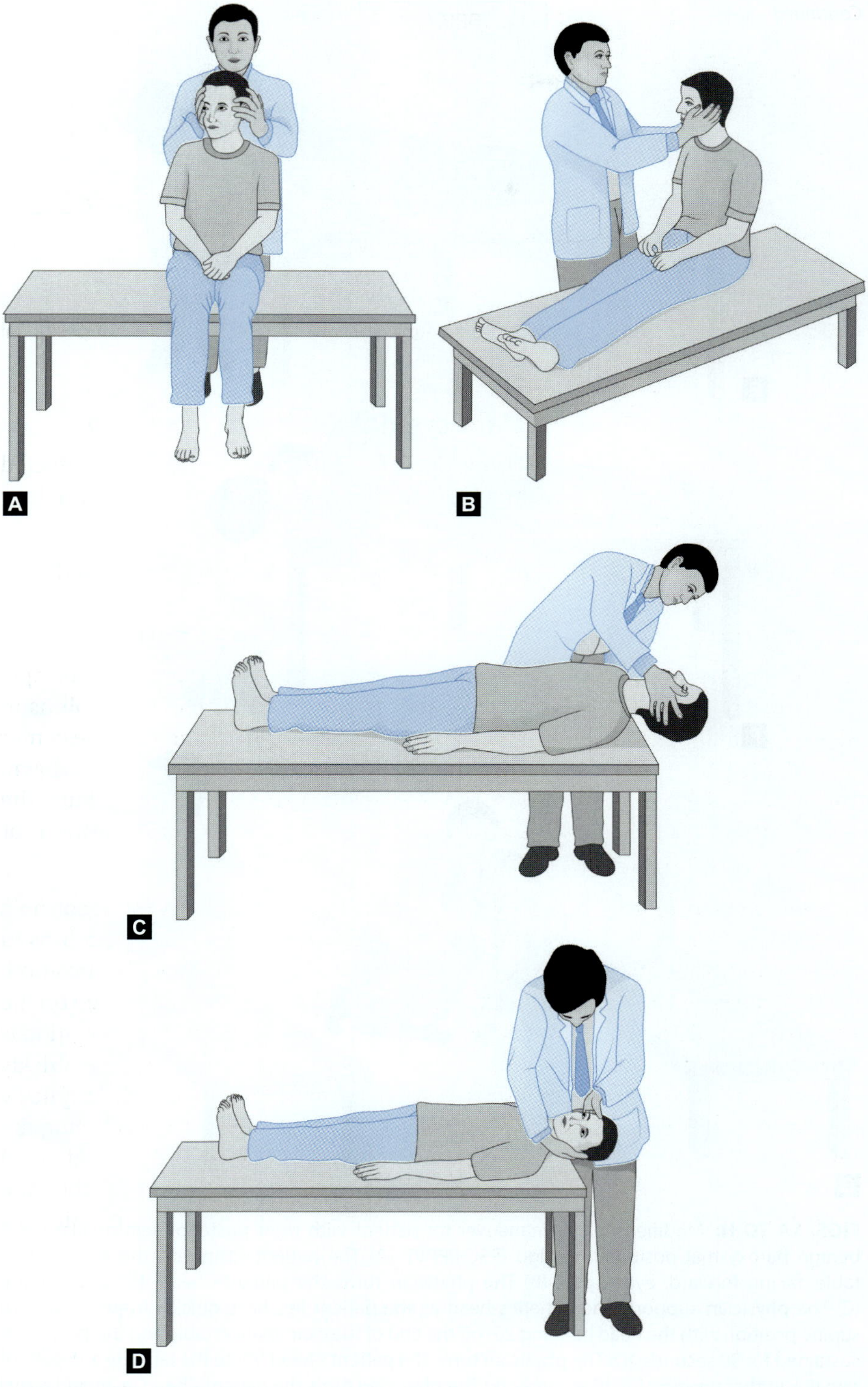

FIGS. 1A TO H: *Continued*

Continued

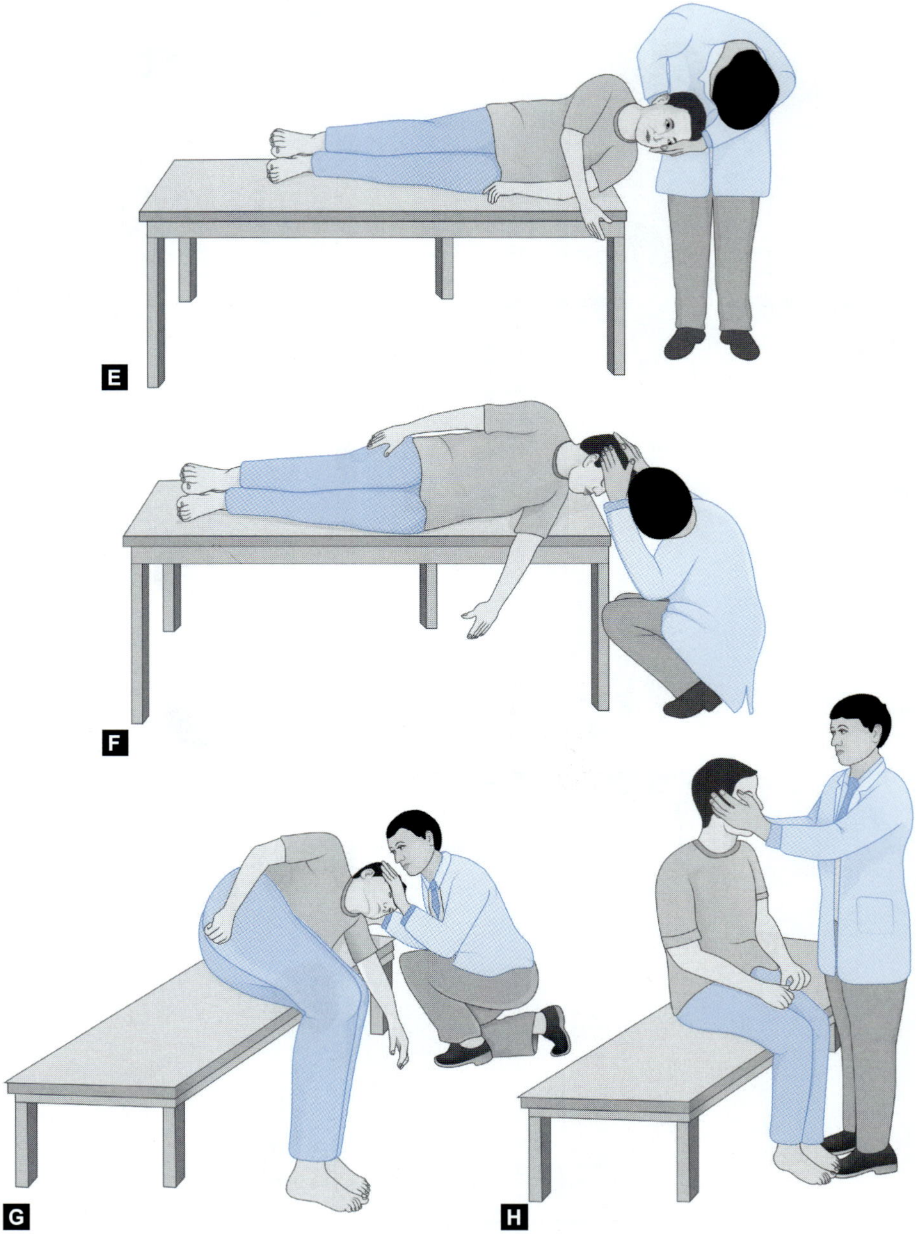

FIGS. 1A TO H: Modified Epley's maneuver for patient with right posterior semicircular canal benign paroxysmal positional vertigo (PSC-BPPV). (A) The patient sitting on the examination table, facing forward, eyes open; (B) The physician turns the patient's head 45° to the right; (C) The physician supports the patient's head as the patient lies back quickly from a sitting to supine position with the head hanging 20° off the end of the examination table and this position is sustained for 30 seconds; (D) The physician turns the patient's head 90° to the left side and patient remains in that position for 30 seconds; (E) The physician turns the patient's head in an additional 90° to the left; (F) While the patient rotates his or her body 90° in the same direction; (G) The patient remains in this position for more than 30 seconds. The patient sits up on the examination table; and (H) Finally, the physician turns the patient's head to the neural position.

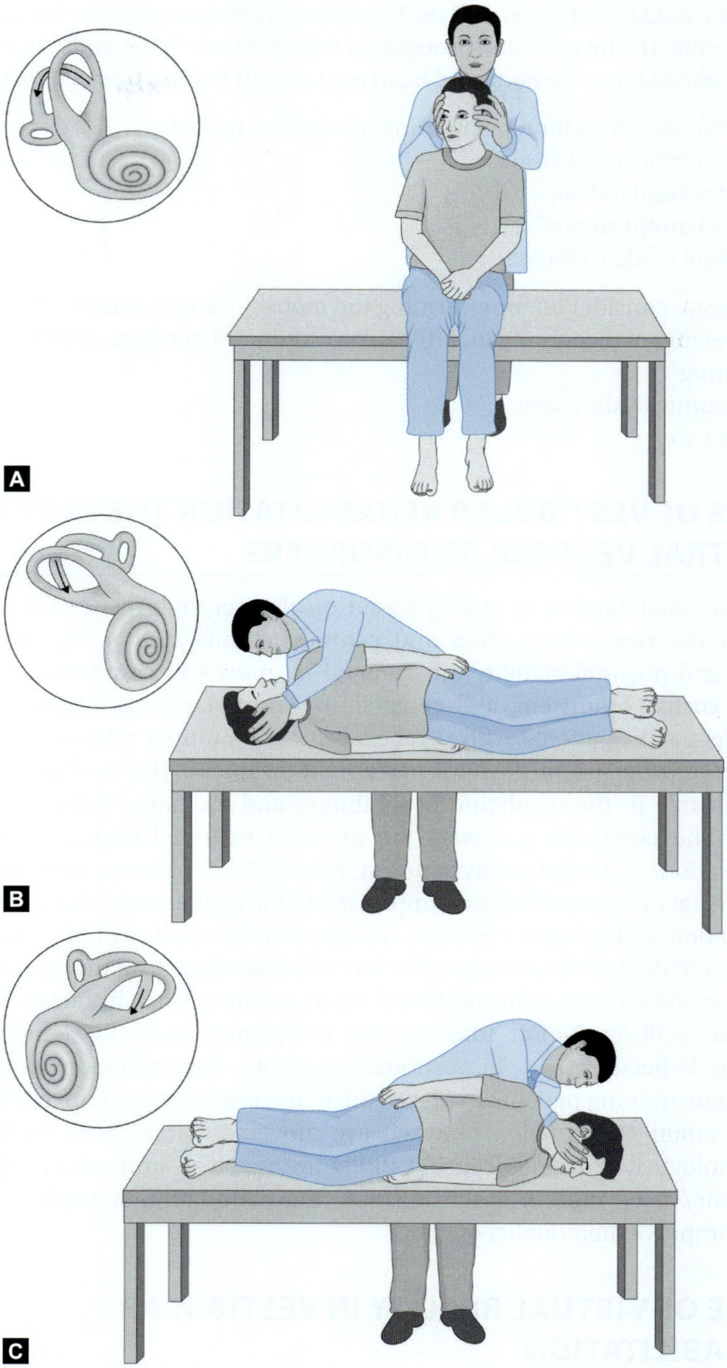

FIGS. 2A TO C: Semont's maneuver. (A) The doctor turns the patient's head so that it is halfway between looking straight ahead and looking away from the side that causes vertigo; (B) the doctor then lowers quickly to the side that causes the vertigo. When the head is on the table, the patient looks up at the ceiling. The patient remains in this position for 30 seconds; and (C) the doctor then quickly moves the patient to the other side of the table without stopping in the upright position. When the head is on the table, the patient looks down at the table. The patient remains in this position for 30 seconds and is then allowed to sit upright.

and is then quickly laid down with the head hanging at an angle of 30° for a duration of 30 seconds. The head is then brought up rapidly to touch the individual's chest, and 30 seconds later, the body and head are brought back to a seated position.

The contraindications for repositioning maneuvers include:

- Severe cervical disc disease
- Vertebrobasilar disease
- Severe carotid stenosis
- Unstable cardiac disease

Few things to consider after performing the repositioning maneuvers:

- Conversion of posterior canal BPPV to anterior or lateral canal BPPV
- Vomiting
- Autonomic dysfunction
- Imbalance

ROLE OF VESTIBULAR REHABILITATION THERAPY IN CENTRAL VESTIBULAR DISORDERS

Vestibular rehabilitation is mainly based on the neuroplasticity and compensation of the vestibular system and central nervous system. Eye-movement stability and postural stability are attained by means of compensation of the cerebral cortex, brainstem, and cerebellum. Vestibular rehabilitation is found to be effective in patients with cerebellar stroke, multiple sclerosis, vestibular migraine, and persistent postural perceptual dizziness. The flocculus plays an important role in the regulation of inhibitory and excitatory branches of VOR pathway and cerebellar pathways are involved in initial stages of vestibular compensation. A recent study showed that 50% of patients with cerebellar infarction have impaired fixation suppression. During the acute phase, vestibular rehabilitation and balance exercises can improve the quality of life. In multiple sclerosis, rehabilitation strategies like saccadic exercises, fixation exercises, and balance exercises may help improve fatigue, balance, and dizziness. Reduced cerebellar VOR inhibition may be the underlying pathophysiology of the vestibular hypersensitivity in vestibular migraine. Rehabilitation in migraine may include training patients to "desensitize" the vestibular system and teaching them to attain coordination between eye movements and head movements. The pathological processes causing PPPD are not well understood. However, optokinetic/visual motion desensitization and habituation strategies can help patients improve their quality of life.

ROLE OF VIRTUAL REALITY IN VESTIBULAR REHABILITATION

The use of virtual reality—both immersive and nonimmersive VR technology for vestibular rehabilitation makes the rehabilitation interesting and more engaging from the patients' side. VR-induced retinal slip creates optokinetic movements, which can enhance mechanisms of adaptation. Virtual reality technology promotes vestibular compensation. Immersive computing environments help in increasing VOR gain. One randomized control trial compared the use of traditional rehabilitation exercises at home (control-group) and the Track Speed Racing 3D-game with a smartphone and head-mounted display (experimental-group) in chronic unilateral vestibular hypofunction. Micarelli et al. reported significant improvement in posturography parameters, VOR gain on the lesional side, as well as Dizziness Handicap Inventory (DHI) and Activities-specific Balance Confidence scale scores in VR group at 4 weeks. Viziano et al. then found that the significant difference remained in the long-term follow-up (56 weeks). The compliance of patients with vestibular rehabilitation was also good in VR-based therapies.

The previous VR approaches were focused on simulating the external reality. A novel technology, sonoception utilizes sound, pressure, and vibration to simulate internal reality. It is a noninvasive technology that provides proprioceptive and vestibular input through a wearable device. This uses vibrotactile transducers to stimulate mechanoreceptors situated on muscles and otolith organs. By stimulating cutaneous receptors on tendons of an immobile limb by using a particular vibration frequency, it generates a sensation of displacement of the immobile limb. Bone-conducted vibration at a particular frequency produces craniocentric whole-body responses, the characteristics of the response being compatible with that of vestibular-mediated responses. The transducers help in turning sound waves into mechanical vibrations, which induce a perception of limb movement and alter the subjects' sense of balance. Sonoception, thus, enables multisensory integration of bodily information and aids in restoring balance.[9]

PRACTICE POINTS IN VESTIBULAR REHABILITATION

- Vestibular rehabilitation therapy should be offered to patients with acute, subacute, and chronic vestibular hypofunction.
- It should be offered to both unilateral and bilateral vestibular disorders.
- Adequate dose should be tailored according to the individual patients.
- Smooth pursuit and saccadic exercises should be offered as a part of vestibular rehabilitation and should never be offered in isolation (i.e., without head movements).
- Whenever feasible, clinician-supervised therapy should be offered to patients as compared to telemedicine, as it increases the adherence to the therapy.
- Age does not affect the potential for improvement. Clinicians should not deny the therapy to older individuals only based on age.
- Sex does not affect the outcome. So, both male and female patients should be treated with expectations for similar results.
- Vestibular rehabilitation therapy is also effective in central vestibular disorders.
- Vestibular rehabilitation has shown to improve patient outcomes regardless of time of onset. However, earlier interventions are preferred.
- Migraine, anxiety, peripheral neuropathy, and long-term use of vestibular suppressants may affect the treatment outcomes.
- Clinicians can use attainment of primary goal, symptom resolution, or plateau in progression as reasons for stopping the rehabilitation therapy.

CONCLUSION

Vestibular rehabilitation forms an effective treatment of peripheral vestibular disorders, and they are promising indications as a treatment for vestibular disorders of central origin. These exercises and maneuvers help reduce the imbalance and prevent falls in these patients. These strategies complement the pharmacotherapy and improve the quality of life.

REFERENCES

1. In Han B. Simplified Vestibular Rehabilitation Therapy. Singapore: Springer Nature; 2022.
2. Whitney SL, Sparto PJ, Furman JM. Vestibular rehabilitation and factors that can affect outcome. Semin Neurol. 2020;40(1):165-72.
3. Hall CD, Herdman SJ, Whitney SL, Anson ER, Carender WJ, Hoppes CW, et al. Vestibular rehabilitation for peripheral vestibular hypofunction: An updated clinical practice guideline from the Academy of Neurologic Physical Therapy of the American Physical Therapy Association. Neurol Phys Ther. 2022;46(2):118-77.
4. Epley JM. The canalith repositioning procedure: For treatment of benign paroxysmal positional vertigo. Otolaryngol Head Neck Surg. 1992;107(3):399-404.
5. Azad T, Pan G, Verma R. Epley maneuver (canalith repositioning) for benign positional vertigo. Acad Emerg Med. 2020;27(7):637-9.
6. Gebhart I, Götting C, Hool SL, Morrison M, Korda A, Caversaccio M, et al. Sémont maneuver for benign paroxysmal positional vertigo treatment: Moving in the correct plane matters. Otol Neurotol. 2021;42(3):e341-7.
7. van den Broek EM, van der Zaag-Loonen HJ, Bruintjes TD. Systematic review: Efficacy of Gufoni maneuver for treatment of lateral canal benign paroxysmal positional vertigo with geotropic nystagmus. Otolaryngol Head Neck Surg. 2014;150(6):933-8.
8. Yang X, Ling X, Shen B, Hong Y, Li K, Si L, et al. Diagnosis strategy and Yacovino maneuver for anterior canal-benign paroxysmal positional vertigo. J Neurol. 2019;266(7):1674-84.
9. Riva G, Serino S, Di Lernia D, Pavone EF, Dakanalis A. Embodied medicine: Mens sana in corpore virtuale sano. Front Hum Neurosci. 2017;11:120.

15

CHAPTER

Surgical Management in Vertigo

Muthukumar Ramamurthy, Sindhu Kalyanaraman

ABSTRACT

Surgical management for vertigo is considered for patients who have debilitating vertigo despite sufficient medical treatment and vestibular rehabilitation. The surgeries are divided into hearing-preserving and hearing-sacrificing procedures. An absolute contraindication for these surgeries is if it is the only hearing ear. For patients with posterior canal benign paroxysmal positional vertigo (BPPV), when medicines and repositioning maneuvers fail, singular neurectomy and posterior canal occlusion can be tried. For patients with Ménière's disease, hearing-preserving procedures like intratympanic steroids, endolymphatic sac procedures, and hearing-sacrificing procedures like labyrinthectomy and vestibular neurectomy are done. In acoustic tumors, various approaches can be used to remove the tumor depending on the location, size, etc. Perilymph fistula and superior semicircular canal defects are grafted or plugged.

INTRODUCTION

Surgical management of vertigo is opted for patients with persistence of intractable symptoms even after exhausting the maximal medical therapy, vestibular rehabilitation, and dietary control. Approximately, 10% of these patients suffering from vertigo may have to be considered for surgical management.[1] The decision for surgery is made bearing in mind many factors such as the hearing level in both ears, frequency and severity of the attacks, subjective level of impairment, and patient compliance and expectations. A thorough preoperative re-evaluation to confirm the diagnosis should be done. Surgery can be divided into hearing-preserving and hearing-destroying procedures. The patient should be well counseled on the procedure, complications, and possible outcomes.

BENIGN PAROXYSMAL POSITIONAL VERTIGO

Benign paroxysmal positional vertigo (BPPV) is the most common vestibular end-organ disorder characterized by brief vertigo induced by typical head movements and it often resolves spontaneously within 6 months of onset or by particle repositioning maneuvers. Surgery is indicated for the small subset of patients with intractable vertigo.

Singular Neurectomy

The singular nerve exits the internal auditory canal (IAC) laterally and courses posteroinferiorly below the round window membrane.

A transmeatal approach under local or general anesthesia is used. After elevation of the tympanomeatal flap, the middle ear is exposed. The round window membrane is visualized. The singular canal is recognized by the white myelinated nerve bundle that runs at an angle to the alignment of the round window membrane. An angled hook is then used to destroy the nerve tissue and the canal is filled with drilled bone dust to prevent regeneration of the nerve.

Successful singular neurectomy is demonstrated by the absence of nystagmus on the Hallpike maneuver on the first postoperative day. Instead, a vertical down beating will be observed for 1–3 days. This will subside after compensatory adaptation process.[2]

Complications

The complications include:
- Injury to cochlea through round window membrane leading sensorineural (SN) loss in 4–41%[3]
- Anatomical variation leading to difficulty in location of singular canal
- Disequilibrium following the surgery may be due to inadequate compensation

As this procedure is technically challenging, posterior semicircular canal (SCC) occlusion is used.[4]

Posterior Semicircular Canal Occlusion

Posterior semicircular canal (PSCC) occlusion creates a closed fluid-filled endolymphatic space between the plug and cupula, both of which are impermeable to endolymph. Thus, the SCC receptors no longer get excited by the otoliths, permanently eliminating the BPPV.

Preliminary cortical mastoidectomy is done through a postaural William Wilde incision. Lateral semicircular canal (LSCC) is identified followed by PSCC **(Fig. 1)**. When the posterior canal otic capsule is identified, the bone is blue-lined. A 3 mm segment of the PSCC is skeletonized. This endosteal island is removed to expose the perilymph. Next, a plug of bone pate is plugged through the fenestra through the PSCC to completely fill the canal **(Fig. 2)**. This leads to intracanalicular ossification. After plugging the canal, the fenestra and surrounding bone are sealed with temporalis fascia and fibrin glue to prevent perilymph leak.

MÉNIÈRE'S DISEASE

Ménière's disease is a disorder of the inner ear that causes severe vertigo, tinnitus, fluctuating hearing loss, and aural fullness. Surgery for patients with Ménière's disease is contemplated for those who have incapacitating vertigo. There are various corrective and destructive procedures. Corrective procedures are done to restore balance and preserve residual hearing. Destructive procedures are done to abolish sensory input from the particular labyrinth, thus in the process destroy hearing as well.

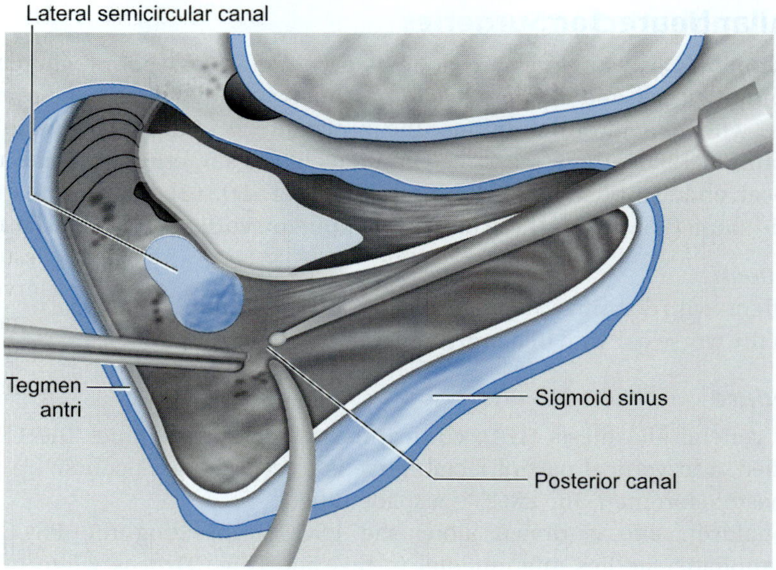

FIG. 1: Identifying the posterior semicircular canal.

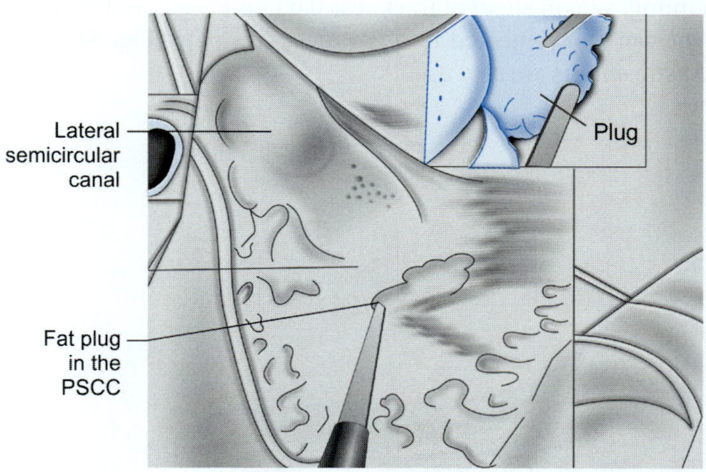

FIG. 2: Plugging the posterior semicircular canal (PSCC).

The choice of surgery depends on:

- *Degree of hearing loss on the affected ear:* Serviceable hearing is defined as pure-tone average (PTA) <50 dB or speech discrimination score (SDS) >50%.[2]
- Severity of the attacks
- Condition of the contralateral ear:
    - Surgery is usually not preferred on the only hearing ear
- Patient age and occupation

Endolymphatic Sac Surgeries

Endolymphatic sac surgeries are done as a corrective procedure whereby the endolymphatic sac and duct are decompressed by removing the bone overlying the sac with or without shunting. The procedure was described initially by Portmann in 1926.[5] There are three variations of sac surgeries done at present: (1) Local endolymphatic sac decompression (LESD), (2) endolymphatic sac mastoid shunt (ESMS), and (3) wide endolymphatic sac decompression (WESD).[6]

Indications:
- Patients with definitive Ménière's who are not responding to medical treatment
- On the worse ear with bilateral Ménière's

Procedure

Under general anesthesia (GA), cortical mastoidectomy is done. The LSCC is identified, and vertical part of facial nerve is traced along its course up to the stylomastoid foramen. The PSCC is also identified.

Donaldson line is drawn along the LSCC transecting the PSCC. The endolymphatic sac lies inferomedial to this line **(Fig. 3)**. It is white in color compared to the gray dura, which is double-folded. The dural plate overlying the endolymphatic sac is removed, exposing the sac. A knife can be used to dissect the outer surface of the sac **(Fig. 4)**. Endolymph escapes from the sac.

For shunting, silicon sheet of thickness 0.05 mm is cut and placed inside the lumen of the sac and projected into the mastoid cavity **(Fig. 5)**. Commercially available Austin shunts are also used.

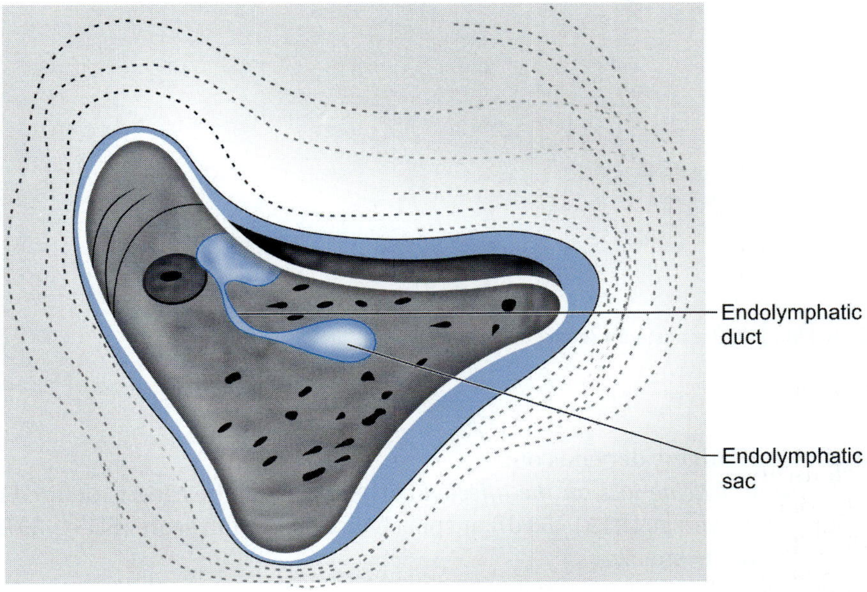

FIG. 3: Endolymphatic sac visualized.

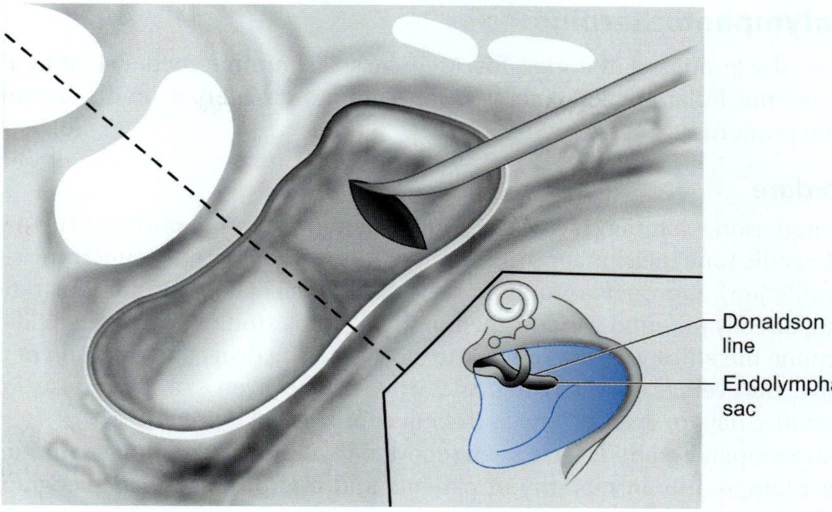

FIG. 4: Endolymphatic sac incised.

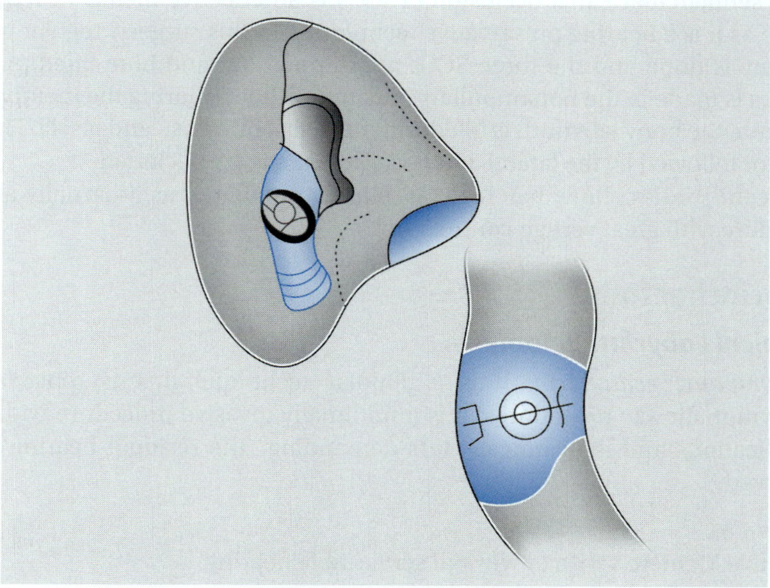

FIG. 5: Endolymphatic shunting.

House modification[7] is the endolymphatic-subarachnoid shunting procedure.

In wide endoscopic skull base surgery (WESD), the posterior and middle fossa including the sigmoid sinus and jugular bulb are exposed, which gives better access to the endolymphatic sac, and thus there is better postoperative vertigo control in severe Ménière's disease.

Intratympanic Steroids

One of the proposed theories for Ménière's is immune-mediated. Steroids decrease the inflammation, increase labyrinthine circulation, and have antioxidant properties.

Procedure

Dexamethasone solution is given through the tympanic membrane (TM) by a small needle (one incision for drug administration and another counter incision for ventilation), as drops via grommet, elevation of the TM flap, and administration of drug directly to round window membrane. Various studies have been made to determine the efficacy of the procedure, dosage of the drug, and duration of the therapy. The average dose is 12 mg/mL, which can be given as a single dose, for 5 consecutive days or even as long as 3–4 injections/year.[8]

Intratympanic steroids have been reported to improve vertiginous symptoms at least temporarily in majority of patients and improve electrocochleography (EcochG).

Triple Semicircular Canal Occlusion

Triple semicircular canal occlusion (TSCO) is an effective means of regulating vertigo as it is a hearing preservative technique.[9] In this surgery, regular mastoidectomy is done and the three SCCs are thinned out and blue lined. A 1 mm fenestra is made in the nonampullary end and without injuring the membranous labyrinth, the bony labyrinth is filled with muscle, bone dust, and fascia. First, the superior followed by the lateral and posterior canals are occluded.

Recent studies show that TSCO is gaining popularity as a partially ablative procedure with great vertigo control rates.

Labyrinthectomy

Chemical Labyrinthectomy

Intratympanic gentamicin: It is a popular technique that is replacing the endolymphatic sac procedures. It is a minimally invasive procedure with fewer complications and is technically less demanding. The residual hearing is also preserved.

Indications:

- Active Ménière's with or without serviceable hearing
- Worse ear in bilateral Ménière's disease
- Tumarkin's otolithic crisis

Intratympanic gentamicin is administered (concentration: 28–40 mg/mL).

The frequency of intratympanic gentamicin administration varies widely. One protocol consists of middle ear installations 3 times a day for 4 days while another entails two intratympanic injections 12 hours apart. Yet another uses a weekly or biweekly schedule.[10]

The titration method of treatment with gaps in between each injection allows for better monitoring for clinical signs of ototoxicity. Treatment must be withheld when the patient develops hearing loss, oscillopsia, and ataxia. Treatment endpoint is when symptomatic control of vertigo is achieved.

Surgical Labyrinthectomy

Transcanal Labyrinthectomy

Transcanal labyrinthectomy is commonly preferred over transmastoid approach as it is less invasive, has a shorter operating time, and has lower morbidity. There is also a direct approach to vestibular end-organ but the surgical exposure is limited. Both approaches are contraindicated when it is in the only hearing ear.

Procedure: An anterior-based tympanomeatal flap is raised. Oval window, round window, stapes footplate, and facial nerve are identified. The incus and stapes are removed. The vestibule may be accessed by enlarging the oval window or connecting the round and oval windows. The five vestibular organs have to be avulsed. The utricle, the lateral and superior SCC is destroyed at the superior aspect. The saccule is damaged by aspiration of the medial aspect into the spherical recess. The neuroepithelium is mechanically probed and removed. Then the vestibule is packed with gel foam and fat tissue.

Postoperative severe vertigo is compensated by central nervous system (CNS) in 1–2 weeks. Vestibular tests are done to ensure that complete ablation has been done.

Transmastoid Labyrinthectomy

The indications for this approach include transcanal labyrinthectomy failures and posttraumatic etiology.

Procedure: A simple mastoidectomy is done and LSCC and PSCC are identified. Labyrinthectomy is done. Both SCCs are opened, and then drilling continued superiorly to common crus and superior SCC **(Fig. 6)**. Then the utricle and saccule are also exposed. The membranous labyrinth is probed with a knife and removed. Fat and muscle plugging are used to seal the defect. Rates of control of vertigo after a transmastoid labyrinthectomy range from 90 to 98%; however, the recurrence of vertigo after a transcanal labyrinthectomy may be as high as 15%.[11]

Vestibular Neurectomy

One of the most effectual means to control disabling vertigo is the denervation of the vestibule, which leads to total vestibular loss in one ear.

Indications:

- Intractable Ménière's disease.
- In patients who have residual hearing, where IT gentamicin or endolymphatic sac procedures have failed; the retrosigmoid or middle cranial fossa approach is done.
- In patients with no hearing, translabyrinthine nerve section can be done.
- Tumarkin's otolithic crisis.

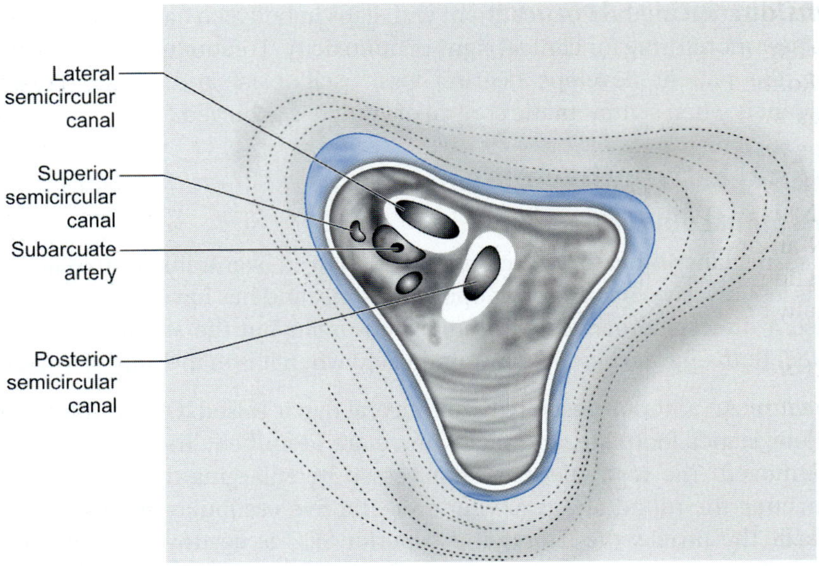

FIG. 6: Three semicircular canals.

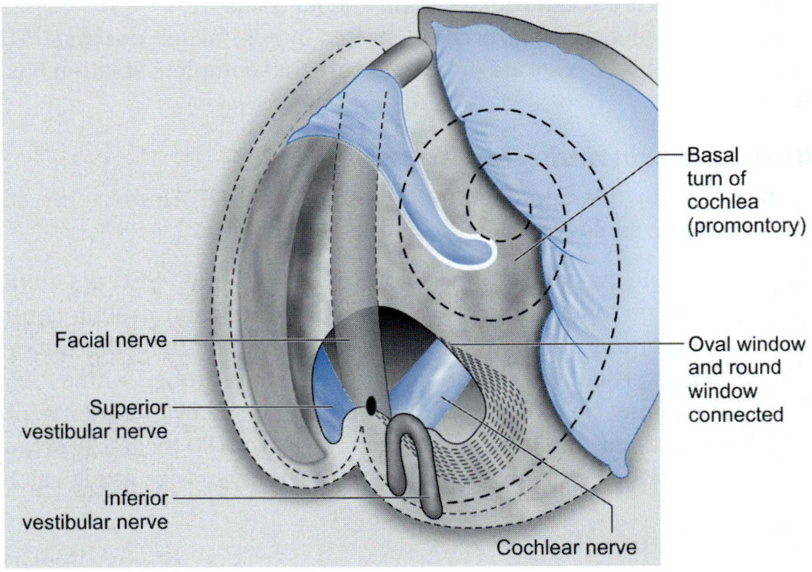

FIG. 7: Structures visualized through the middle ear.

Transmeatal Approach

The transmeatal operation provides the most direct anatomical route to the internal auditory canal. It may be indicated in advanced unilateral Ménière's disease with very poor hearing and poststapedectomy vertigo.

A tympanomeatal flap is raised, the round and oval windows are connected, cochlear and vestibule are opened widely. Then the IAC and its neuromuscular bundle are identified. The facial nerve is situated anterosuperiorly and the cochlear nerve lies inferior to it **(Fig. 7)**. The vestibular nerve lies posteriorly and is sectioned.

Translabyrinthine Approach

This approach is done in patients with no serviceable hearing.

Routine mastoidectomy is done and mastoid antrum LSCC, short process of incus and facial nerve are identified. Labyrinthectomy is done. The IAC is accessed at the vestibule by blue lining over it. The lateral aspect of IAC is skeletonized. The proper identification of the nerves should be done. The superior vestibular nerve (SVN) is sharply demarcated from the facial nerve, which lies deep into it. The SVN and the inferior vestibular nerve (IVN) are sectioned proximal to Scarpa's ganglion. Facial nerve should be monitored to avoid injury. The cochlear nerve is usually preserved for future cochlear implants.[12]

Retrolabyrinthine Approach

The retrolabyrinthine approach offers excellent exposure of the cerebellopontine (CP) angle with little morbidity.

Under GA, an extended mastoidectomy is done so as to expose endolymphatic sac. The posterior fossa is accessed through a window created surgically bounded by facial nerve anteriorly, sigmoid sinus posteriorly, middle fossa superiorly, and the jugular bulb inferiorly. The dura is incised and cerebrospinal fluid (CSF) is drained.

The vestibular nerve can normally be found 2 cm deep to the point at which the PSCC bisects the vertical facial nerve. The vestibular and cochlear segments are separated, and the vestibular portion is sectioned with a sharp knife. Dura is closed with temporalis facia and wound is closed in layers.

Retrosigmoid Approach

Retrosigmoid approach is one of the most commonly used procedures because of the short operating time and ease. It provides the maximum exposure of the CP angle contents.

The retrosigmoid approach begins with a postauricular incision and then, posterior craniotomy is done, CSF is released, and cerebellum is retracted. Then, the CP angle is visualized. IAC is then identified laterally and bone over superior, posterior, and inferior parts is drilled.

The dura of the IAC is incised along its long axis and vestibular nerves are identified. The SVN and singular nerve is cut while the inferior vestibular nerve is preserved due to its proximity to the cochlear nerve. The dura is closed and wound is closed in layers.

A recent advance is the use of endoscope to visualize the IAC contents. This provides a better magnification and precise sectioning of both vestibular nerves.

Middle Cranial Fossa Approach

The middle cranial fossa approach allows the selective resection of the meatal segment of the vestibular nerve.

Under GA, a pretragal incision is made. The temporalis muscle is divided into five flaps **(Fig. 8)**.

A 2 × 3 cm craniotomy is made, and temporal lobe is retracted. The dura is elevated from the floor up to the arcuate eminence and bone of IAC. The facial

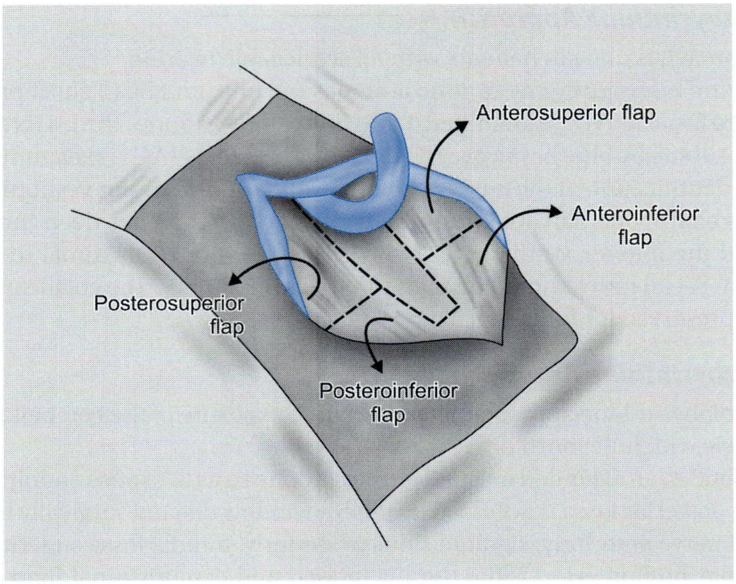

FIG. 8: Five flaps of the temporalis muscle.

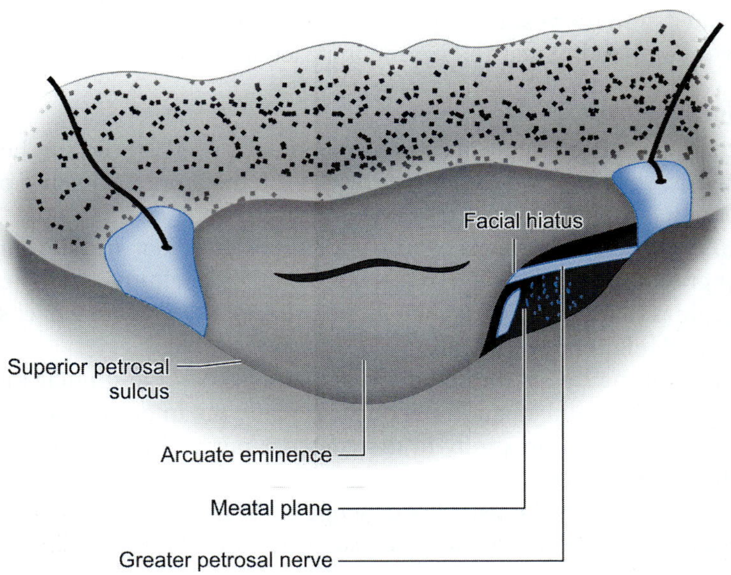

FIG. 9: Facial hiatus in the middle cranial fossa extradural approach.

hiatus [point of exit of greater superficial petrosal nerve (GSPN)] is visualized **(Fig. 9)**. The bone over the arcuate eminence is drilled exposing the labyrinth. The blue lining of the superior canal is identified. The GSPN is identified up to the geniculate ganglion.

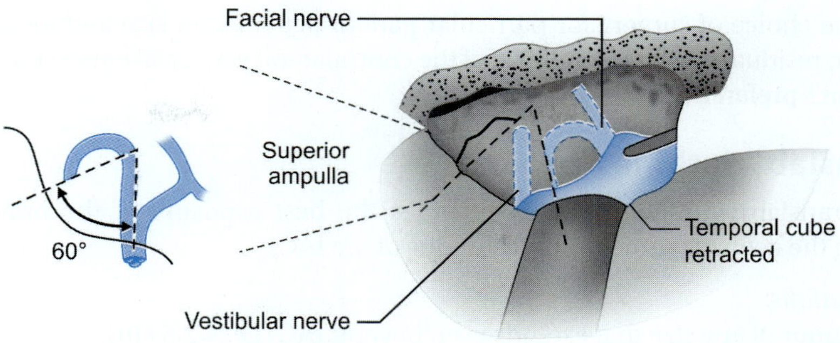

FIG. 10: Identifying the sac internal auditory canal.

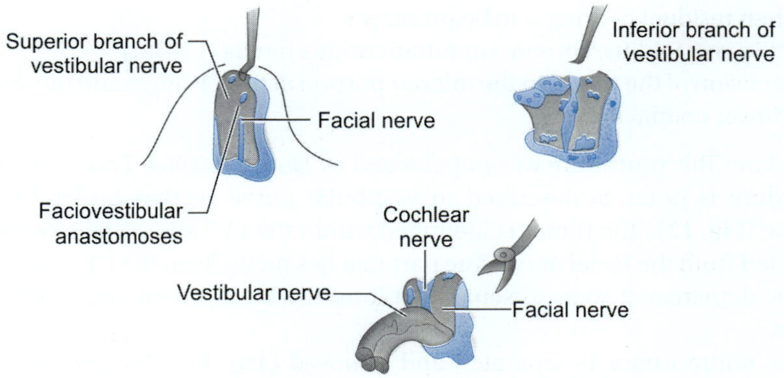

FIG. 11: Resection of the vestibular nerve in the inferior cerebellar artery.

The IAC can be identified by three methods.[1] A line drawn 60° from the superior canal identifies the IAC or it can be identified at the porus and followed laterally till the geniculate ganglion **(Fig. 10)**. Another method is to follow the GSPN to the geniculate ganglion thereby locating the IAC fundus. The bill's bar serves as a landmark for IAC fundus.

The contents of the IAC are demarcated individually. The vestibular nerve along with the singular nerve and Scarpa's ganglion is cut **(Fig. 11)**.

Miscellaneous

Sham surgery is performing a simple mastoidectomy for patients with vertigo. Thomsen et al.,[13] in a Danish study, reported a better success rate as compared to sac procedures. Benefits of these miscellaneous procedures remain controversial.

ACOUSTIC NEUROMA

This is a benign tumor that arises from the Schwann cells of the vestibular nerve.

Principle:
- Complete removal of tumor
- Reduction of mortality
- Preservation of facial nerve and cochlear nerve

The choice of surgery for particular patient depends on size and location of tumor, residual hearing, condition of the contralateral ear, facial nerve status, and patient's preference.

Translabyrinthine Approach

The translabyrinthine approach provides the best exposure of the brainstem facing the acoustic tumor and the fundus of the IAC.

Indications:
- Tumor of any size that extends even beyond IAC (i.e., >2.5 cm)
- No serviceable hearing present
- When the facial nerve is involved and the entire nerve is to be traced

Contraindications:
- When residual hearing is to be preserved
- Active mastoiditis/chronic suppurative otitis media (CSOM)
- Extension of the tumor in the inferior portion of the CP angle and involvement of lower cranial nerves

Procedure: This procedure was popularized by House in 1964. Translabyrinthine procedure is done as described in vestibular nerve section under Ménière's disease **(Fig. 12)**. The tumor is identified within the IAC and should be carefully dissected from the facial nerve. The part that lies medially in the CP angle should also be demarcated so as to separate it from the brain steam and other cranial nerves.

The entire tumor is separated and removed **(Fig. 13)**. The fifth and lower cranial nerves and the vessels are preserved as much as possible. The dural defects are closed with abdominal fat and fascia. Wound is closed in layers.

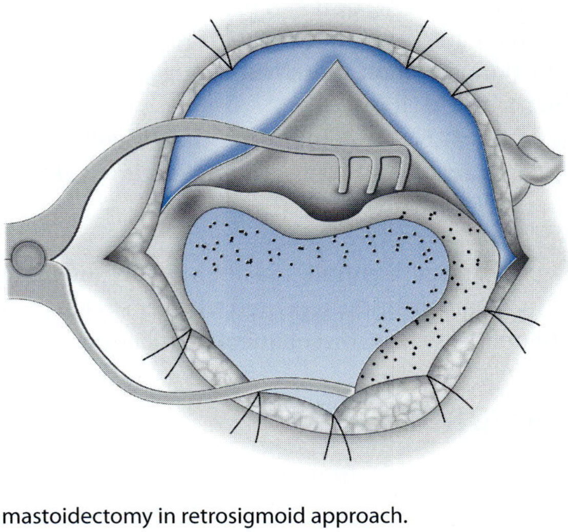

FIG. 12: Extended mastoidectomy in retrosigmoid approach.

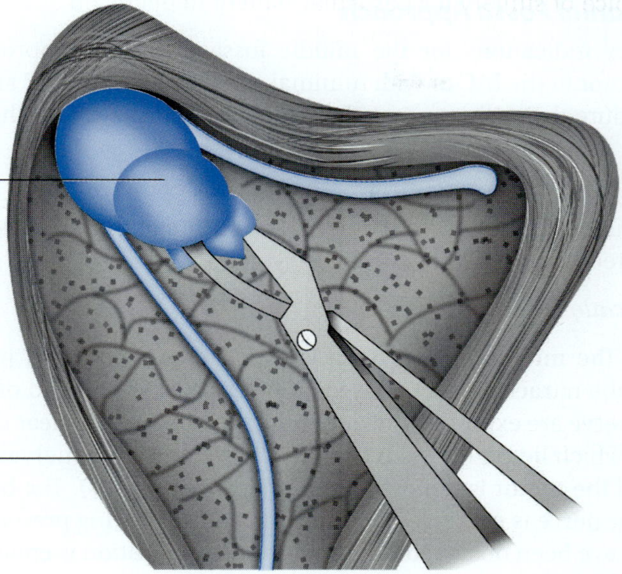

FIG. 13: Tumor removal.

Retrosigmoid Approach

The retrosigmoid approach can be used for small to large tumors that occupy the CP angle and internal auditory meatus (IAM) except the far lateral portion of the internal artery canal. It provides a best panoramic view of the posterior fossa with hearing preservation.

Indications:
- Tumor of any size, especially if located in inferior portion of CP angle
- Residual hearing to be preserved
- Revision surgery

Contraindications: More than 2 cm lateral extension into IAC or extension into cranial base.

Procedure: As in the vestibular neurectomy, retrosigmoid area is approached. The CP angle and IAC exposed. Anterior inferior cerebellar artery (AICA) and posterior inferior cerebellar artery (PICA) identified. The bone over superior, posterior, and inferior parts of the IAC is drilled. The dura of the IAC is incised along its long axis.

At this stage the tumor is identified. The dissection is first done between tumor and facial nerve. The tumor and the eighth nerve are transected above the plane and the intracanalicular portion is removed. The CP angle portion of the tumor is first debulked by making an incision over surface of tumor. Intracapsular debulking is done using cavitron ultrasonic surgical aspirator (CUSA) or Laser.[14] Then the capsule is very carefully separated by microdissection.

Middle Cranial Fossa Approach

The primary indications for the middle fossa extradural approach are small acoustic tumor in the IAC or with minimal extension into the CP angle as it is the only procedure that fully exposes the lateral third of the IAC without sacrificing hearing.

Indications:

- Small tumors in the IAC with minimal extension in the CP angle.
- Good preoperative hearing.

Contraindication: Large tumors > 2 cm.

Procedure: The middle cranial fossa is exposed as mentioned previously. The temporal lobe retracted and IAC is identified. At the lateral end of IAC, bill's bar and facial nerve are exposed. The dura is further divided for clear demarcation of the tumor, which lies in between the vestibular nerves. The nerves are sectioned distally and the tumor is removed from the canal **(Fig. 14)**. The blood supply of the cochlear nerve is preserved. In this procedure, hearing preservation rates of up to 70% have been observed. An important complication is epilepsy due to the temporal lobe retraction.

Recurrence is uncommon after acoustic tumor removal (recurrence <5%).

PERILYMPH FISTULA

Perilymph fistula (PLF) is a condition resulting from abnormal connection between the inner ear perilymph and middle ear space. The surgical procedure is exploratory tympanotomy, which involves locating the site of leak and grafting of the fistula.

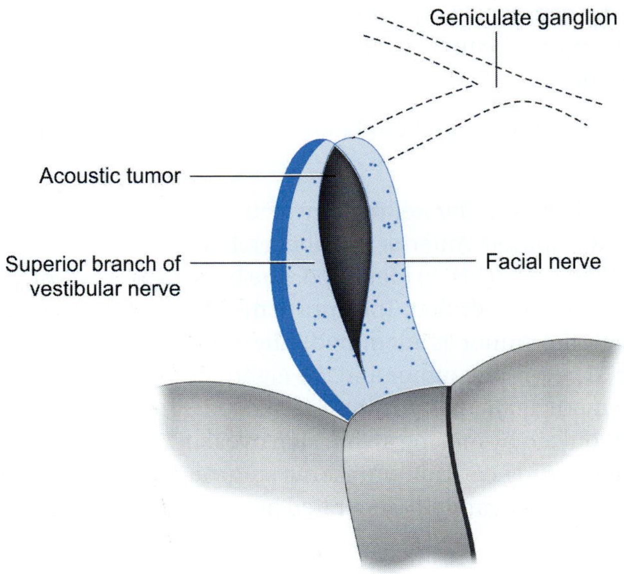

FIG. 14: Acoustic neuroma excision.

Surgery is considered if the hearing deteriorates or the vestibular symptoms fail to abate even after 4 weeks of conservative management.

Perilymph Fistula Following Stapedectomy (Surgery for Otosclerosis)

The PLF is one of the common causes of sensorineural hearing loss (SNHL) following stapedectomy.

There are two types:

1. Primary or early perilymph fistula, which occurs immediately after surgery.
2. Secondary or delayed PLF.

Procedure: Under local anesthesia, tympanomeatal flap is elevated and the middle ear is entered. Leak site is looked for. If not found, patient placed in Trendelenburg position by tilting the table and Valsalva maneuver is done. The fluid now collected is tested for glucose and protein. The most common site of the leak is at the oval window anterior or below the anterior crus. A temporalis fascia graft is placed over the leak and packed in place with gel foam.

In cases of round window trauma, the tear is visible around the annular ring. A clot or granulation tissue is occasionally found around the leak. The defect is repaired with tragal perichondrium.

For poststapedectomy PLF, the fistulous tract is excised, and prosthesis is removed. A soft tissue is used to seal the fenestra and prosthesis is kept over it. Hearing improvement is only minimal after surgery but vertigo and tinnitus usually resolve. Thus, early diagnosis and intervention are mandatory.

About 72–90% of the patient report significant improvement of vertigo. Hearing improvement has been reported in 13–49% while deterioration of hearing in 11–17% of patients has been reported.[15]

SUPERIOR SEMICIRCULAR CANAL DEHISCENCE

Superior semicircular canal dehiscence (SSCD) is a relatively new condition which was first described by Minor in 1998.[16] It is the absence of the bone overlying the superior SCC causing a third window. Conservative treatment for SSCD is used for patients with mild symptoms. A tympanostomy tube may be tried with variable symptom relief.

Surgical treatment of SSCD (bony dehiscence is resurfaced, plugged, or capped) is considered for patients who exhibit severe incapacitating symptoms. The two main approaches are the transmastoid and the middle fossa craniotomy approach to close the dehiscence.

Resurfacing includes dural elevation over arcuate eminence to avoid damage to membranes and dehiscence is either closed with fascia and bone dust.

Plugging is done by complete occlusion of the superior canal by bone pate.

Round window plugging is a recent advance for control of hyperacusis in SSCD.[17]

VESTIBULAR PAROXYSMIA

Neurovascular cross-compression of the root entry zone of the eighth cranial nerve may cause local demyelination and axonal hyperactivity resulting in typical paroxysmal vestibular and/or cochlear symptoms. The AICA or PICA or a vein may cause neural compression which causes disabling positional vertigo. Carbamazepine is the drug of choice with a good control of the symptoms in most of the patients. Those patients not responding to carbamazepine may be candidates for microvascular decompression surgery.[18]

CONCLUSION

Surgical procedures for patients with vertigo are infrequently done nowadays. With the better understanding of the pathophysiological mechanisms and advent of improved medical therapies and minimally invasive techniques like intratympanic gentamicin treatment, which give equal or sometimes even better symptomatic relief, surgeries are falling out of use. However, surgeries for specific indications, in selective patients, can give excellent results.

REFERENCES

1. Adunka OF, Buchman CA. Otology, Neurotology, and Lateral Skull Base Surgery. India: Thieme. 2011. pp. 353-5.
2. Brackmann DE. Cough shelton. In: Arriaga MA (Ed). Otologic Surgeries, 3rd edition. Philadelphia: Saunders Elsevier; 2010. pp. 466-7, 581-9.
3. Crane BT, Crey JP, Minor LB. Glasscock-Shambaugh Surgery of the Ear, 6th edition. Connecticut (USA): PMPH; 2010. pp. 563-81.
4. Leveque M, Labrousse M, Seidermann L, Chays A. Surgical therapy in intractable benign paroxysmal positional vertigo. Otolaryngol Head Neck Surg. 2007;136(5):693-8.
5. Portmann G. The saccus endolymphaticus and an operation for draining the same for the relief of vertigo. J Laryngol Otol. 1991;105(12):1109-12.
6. Zheng G, Liu Y, He J, Li S, Zhang Q, Duan M, et al. A Comparison of local endolymphatic sac decompression, endolymphatic mastoid shunt, and wide endolymphatic sac decompression in the treatment of intractable Meniere's disease: A short-term follow-up investigation. Front Neurol. 2022;13:810352.
7. House WF. Subarachnoid shunt for drainage of endolymphatic hydrops. Laryngoscope. 1962;72:713-29.
8. Bolease MS, Santina CD, Minor LM. Longitudinal results with intratympanic dexamethasone in the treatment of Meniere's disease. Abstract of the American Neurotology Society; 2007.
9. Tian J, Yin G, Zhang Q, Zhang S, Zeng X, Li Y. Triple semicircular canal occlusion with endolymphatic sac decompression for intractable Meniere's disease. Front Neurol. 2024;15:1362603.
10. Hain TC. Dizziness-and-balance.com. (2024). Intratympanic/transtympanic gentamicin treatment for Meniere's Disease. [online] Available from www.dizziness-and-balance.com/treatment/ttg.html [Last accessed April, 2025].
11. Huang TC, Levine SC. (2015). Transmastoid and transcanal labyrinthectomy. In: Middle Ear and Mastoid Surgeries. [online] Available from https://entokey.com/transmastoid-and-transcanal-labyrinthectomy/ [Last accessed April, 2025].
12. Teufert KB, Doherty J. Endolymphatic sac shunt, labyrinthectomy, and vestibular nerve section in Meniere's disease. Meniere's disease. Otolaryngol Clin N Am. 2010;43(5):1090-111.

13. Thomsen J, Bonding P, Becker B, Stage J, Tos M. The non-specific effect of endolymphatic sac surgery in treatment of Meniere's disease: a prospective, randomized controlled study comparing "classic" endolymphatic sac surgery with the insertion of a ventilating tube in the tympanic membrane. Acta Otolaryngol. 1998;118:769-3.
14. Packer MD, Bradley WD. Vestibular schwannoma. In: Glasscock-Shambaugh. Surgery of the ear, 6th edition. Connecticut (USA): PMPH; 2010. pp. 643-83.
15. Kutz Jr JW. Roland PS. Medscape. (2022). Perilymphatic fistula treatment & management. [online]. Available from www.emedicine.medscape.com/article/856806-treatment#d15 [Last accessed April, 2025].
16. Minor LB, Slomon D, Zinreich J, Zee DS. Sound-and/or pressure-induced vertigo due to bone dehiscence of the superior semicircular canal. Arch Otolaryngol Head Neck Surg. 1998;124:249-58.
17. Nikkar-Esfahani A, Whelan D, Banerjee A. Occlusion of the round window: A novel way to treat hyperacusis symptoms in superior semicircular canal dehiscence syndrome. J Laryngol Otol. 2013;127(7):705-7.
18. Thomas Brandt. Vertigo-Its Multisensory Syndromes. New Delhi: Springer. 2013;1:117-25.

16 CHAPTER Definition and Approach to Syncope

Vivek Mathew

ABSTRACT

Syncope is a symptom with transient loss of consciousness due to transient global cerebral hypoperfusion. On one hand, the most common cause for this is neurally mediated neurocardiogenic syncope, which does not alter the long-term morbidity. On the other side of the spectrum are the cardiac arrhythmias, some of which can be precursors to sudden cardiac death if not treated adequately. This chapter provides an overview and an approach to a patient presenting with symptoms resembling syncope to the emergency.

INTRODUCTION

Syncope is a symptom and is defined as transient loss of consciousness (TLOC) due to global cerebral hypoperfusion (GCHP).[1] It is one of the causes for TLOC, where the term transient refers to short duration with spontaneous and complete recovery. The time duration for "short" or "transient" has not been specified but is generally less than a few minutes. By definition, the cause for TLOC has to be cerebral hypoperfusion and global rather than focal. The patient would, of course, present with history of TLOC and the subject of this chapter is the process of coning down (see list of sequential questions given later in this chapter). Patients and families often assume that since they lost consciousness, they need to meet a neurologist; however, sinister causes of syncope lie in the domain of the cardiologist or the cardiac electrophysiologist. The importance of evaluation for syncope also lies in these sinister causes, where syncope could actually be a harbinger of sudden cardiac death (SCD).

Presyncope is the term used for the prodromal symptoms in isolation without loss of consciousness or fall. These symptoms are usually stereotyped and consist of light-headedness, giddiness, and may be associated with graying of vision, sweating, and fatigue.

SEQUENTIAL QUESTIONS TO BE ANSWERED

- Was there really TLOC or was consciousness preserved during the fall?
- If there was TLOC, is the mechanism related to perfusion or other mechanisms?
- If apparently related to perfusion, was it global or was there focal hypoperfusion or ischemia?
- If there was GCHP, what was the mechanism for it?
  - Was it due to a primary cardiac problem (arrhythmia or structural cardiac abnormality)?
  - Was it neurally mediated abnormality of blood pressure and cerebral perfusion maintaining reflex mechanisms (neurocardiogenic syncope)?
  - Was it due to an inability to maintain adequate blood pressure in the standing position (orthostatic hypotension)?

APPROACH

History

History of Events

A patient with transient loss of consciousness reporting to the clinic requires time, and most of the time goes into detailed history. Each episode of syncope that has occurred needs to be noted down along with source of history. At times, this may necessitate calling up a relative on phone to clarify some details. At the end of history, to the extent possible, we should be able to mentally visualize the circumstances and setting for each episode that the patient has had. This would give us information on the setting, preictal, ictal, and postictal events.

Past History

Any history of cardiac or neurological illness should be probed for. Family history of SCD should be specifically asked for.

Physical Examination

The physical examination includes search for pallor, edema, pulse rate and volume, peripheral and carotid pulse, blood pressure in supine and standing position, blood pressure in both arms and legs and cardiac and neurological examination including a review of autonomic functions.

Laboratory Tests

History and examination will determine if blood counts, renal functions, serum albumin, thyroid stimulating hormone, urine protein, or any other laboratory tests are needed.

Electrocardiogram

Electrocardiogram (ECG) is mandatory for every patient coming with history of possible syncope. A careful examination of the ECG with or without rhythm strip can give clues to underlying arrhythmogenic disorders or structural abnormalities. The morphology of the QRS complex can give indications for accessory pathways; measurement of the segments can give clues to presence of cardiac channel disorders like long-QT syndrome and Brugada syndrome. Presence of ventricular ectopics can suggest underlying cardiac disease.

Echocardiography

Cardiac echocardiography is required for those patients where history, examination, or ECG point to the possibility of an underlying structural abnormality of the heart. This can pick up valvular heart disease, left ventricular outflow obstruction, regional wall motion abnormalities, right ventricular dysplasia, etc. The presence of these abnormalities does not directly mean that these are the cause of the patient's symptoms.

Electrophysiological Tests

Cardiac electrophysiological tests are required in those where arrhythmias are suspected on basis of history and examination. Structurally damaged hearts are also more prone to arrhythmias. Some disorders can be picked up on 24 hours (up to 48 hours) by Holter monitoring; however, the yield is less when the events are infrequent. The presence of frequent ventricular ectopics or nonsustained ventricular tachycardia would not be diagnostic in itself but would indicate need for further cardiac evaluation. Some patients will require cardiac catheterization with electrophysiological studies including stimulation. Finally, some with very occasional episodes but higher index of suspicion for an arrhythmia will need an implantable loop recorder, which can monitor events for several months (6–18 months) at a time.[2] Interpretation of results of cardiac catheterization and implantable loop recorders would be done by cardiologists with interest in cardiac electrophysiology.

Miscellaneous

The head-up tilt-table test (HUTT) can be done both with and without drug (usually a nitrate). This test helps to examine the neural reflexes maintaining blood pressure, and thus cerebral perfusion. The patient needs to be fasting for 2 hours prior. Some patients will be on drugs that influence the cardiac or autonomic system. These are often implicated as contributing factors for the syncope and thus need not be stopped prior to HUTT. The patient lies supine for 30–45 minutes and then in 60–80° tilt for another 30–45 minutes. Echocardiogram is monitored continuously. Blood pressure is also preferably monitored continuously with noninvasive digital plethysmography being popular.[3] There have been discussions on the practical utility of HUTT. In patients with high clinical index of suspicion for neurocardiogenic syncope, the HUTT does not add any information to change the algorithm. If the history were typical, the diagnosis would remain neurocardiogenic, even if the HUTT is negative. On the other hand, when the index of suspicion is low, a positive HUTT does not mean that all the previous episodes were neurocardiogenic unless the patient is able to categorically say that the symptoms during HUTT were exactly the same as all previous episodes. Tilt-table testing is avoided in patients with hemodynamically significant stenosis in the cerebral circulation, recent stroke or transient ischemic attack (TIA), proximal coronary artery stenosis, critical mitral stenosis, and clinically significant left ventricular outflow stenosis.

Carotid sinus massage can trigger syncope. The European Society of Cardiology in 2009 recommended that all patients over 40 years of age with history suggestive of syncope and with initial negative evaluation should be taken up for carotid sinus massage for 10 seconds on both sides, in both supine and standing positions (thus, often combined with HUTT).[4] It should be avoided in patients with history of TIA or stroke within the last 3 months, or with carotid bruit or documented carotid stenosis on previous Doppler.

Neurological Studies

Neurological studies like imaging (of brain or cerebral vessels) and electro-encephalography (EEG) are not indicated unless history suggests that the falls could be related to either focal cerebral hypoperfusion or that the events themselves are seizures. It needs to be kept in mind that syncope prolonged for more than 1 minute or so could be associated with tonic posturing or a few clonic twitches (convulsive syncope) and also that tongue bite at the tip of the tongue occurs more often during fall in syncope. Tongue bite during tonic phase of generalized seizures tends to be on the lateral aspect of the tongue. Very rarely, seizures can be associated with arrhythmias, for example, temporal or insular seizures causing ictal bradyarrhythmia or asystole. This can be reliably diagnosed only if an ictus is captured during prolonged video-EEG monitoring along with ECG leads.

DIFFERENTIAL DIAGNOSIS

Falls without Loss of Consciousness

Falls without loss of consciousness need to be differentiated from syncope. Fall without loss of consciousness can occur in drop attacks due to atonic or myoclonic seizures or in craniovertebral junction anomalies. Drop attacks of uncertain pathophysiology occur in young women as well. Drop attacks can occur in peripheral vestibular dysfunction as well (e.g., Tumarkin's otolithic crisis in Méniére's disease). These are usually associated with a sensation of being pushed.[5]

Differentials for Transient Loss of Consciousness

Patients with syncope will have a TLOC. It could be very brief lasting only a few seconds. Thus, the patients may say that they remember the preceding and subsequent events well. The question to ask is if they remembers the fall itself. Falls with loss of consciousness can also occur in:

- Generalized tonic-clonic seizures (not related to cerebral perfusion) or posterior circulation ischemia (related to focal cerebral hypoperfusion rather than global). Detailed history of ictus will help to differentiate, other times prolonged video telemetry EEG capturing an ictus would be needed to establish seizures as the cause for the TLOC.

- Posterior circulation TIAs will most often cause other symptoms like double vision, slurring of speech, or imbalance.
- Sudden and transient loss of consciousness can occur in subarachnoid hemorrhage, but the patient will usually wake up with a severe headache and have neck stiffness on examination. A plain computed tomography (CT) brain scan will establish diagnosis.
- Sudden loss of consciousness can also occur rarely with massive pulmonary embolism. Chest and respiratory symptoms will tend to dominate when the patient regains consciousness.[6]

Differential Diagnosis of Syncope

Syncope itself can be precipitated by three different mechanisms:

1. Neurocardiogenic syncope
2. Cardiac causes of syncope
3. Orthostatic hypotension

Neurocardiogenic Syncope

Neurocardiogenic syncope is the most common cause of syncope and least sinister.[7] Other terms used for this are vasovagal syncope. In typical cases, the diagnosis is established on history itself, and if the history is typical and examination and ECG are normal, further testing is not necessary. A typical history would be of long duration (often childhood-onset) but of very occasional symptoms, with falls always happening from sitting or standing position, with precipitating factors like standing for long time, sudden pain, emotionally intense situations, and seeing blood or in anticipation or related to micturition.

The pathophysiology is sudden reduction of heart rate or blood pressure resulting in GCHP. The failure of reflex mechanisms for maintaining blood pressure and heart rate can occur at central and/or peripheral levels. This happens with venous pooling, relative central hypovolemia, and resultant inappropriate sympathetic withdrawal (leading to peripheral vasodilatation, thus causing hypotension), and/or parasympathetic (vagal) stimulation (leading to bradycardia or transient asystole). This can be simulated in the clinical laboratory using HUTT, as previously described. The HUTT test is said to be positive if both symptoms (syncope or presyncope) and hemodynamic changes (hypotension and/or bradycardia) occur. Isolated hemodynamic changes without symptoms are not specific.

Depending on the HUTT results, neurocardiogenic syncope is classified into three types **(Table 1)**.

This classification does not hold for cases where there is excessive rise in heart rate beyond 130 beats/min or where carotid sinus hypersensitivity is demonstrated.[3] Occurrence of symptoms without hemodynamic changes is suggestive of psychogenic syncope. Some centers use “drug tilt” protocols (usually nitrates) as venodilators to increase the peripheral venous pooling and trigger a syncope.

TABLE 1: Types of neurocardiogenic syncope on basis of head-up tilt table test findings.[3]

Type	Also known as	Heart rate	Blood pressure
1	Mixed	During syncope ≥40 beats/min or falls to <40 beats/min for <10 sec ± asystole <3 seconds	Falls prior to fall in heart rate
2A	Cardioinhibitory	During syncope, falls to <40 beats/min for >10 seconds ± asystole >3 seconds	Falls prior to fall in heart rate
2B	Cardioinhibitory	During syncope, falls to <40 beats/min for >10 sec ± asystole >3 seconds	Falls to <80 mm Hg systolic at or after rapid fall in heart rate
3	Pure vasodepressor	During syncope, does not fall >10% from its peak	Fall in blood pressure precipitates syncope

Situational syncopes—some individuals have neurally mediated reflex syncope in specific situations. One example of this is micturition syncope. Others are post-tussive (cough syncope) and those associated with swallowing or defecation.

Carotid sinus hypersensitivity can be an occasional cause for syncope especially in elderly (older persons wearing tight collars and looking up as might happen if visiting the Sistine Chapel or Golden Gate in formal dress). The carotid sinus contains baroreceptors, which can trigger both vagal activation and sympathetic inhibition. Increased sensitivity of the carotid sinus can occur in older individuals.

Cardiac Causes of Syncope

While these are less common, they are the most sinister. Some of them are precursors to SCD. Cardiac causes can be classified into two broad groups:

1. Cardiac arrhythmias
2. Structural abnormalities of the heart, with or without secondary arrhythmias.

Cardiac Arrhythmias

Patients with Wolff-Parkinson-White syndrome (accessory pathways), or with cardiac channelopathies like long-QT syndrome or Brugada syndrome need to be identified as these could be causes for SCD in younger individuals. The channelopathies are often familial, and this underlies the importance of taking history of SCD. Some structural abnormalities are sinister due to their propensity for arrhythmias. An example of this is arrhythmogenic right ventricular dysplasia, also known as arrhythmogenic right ventricular cardiomyopathy, which predisposes to ventricular tachycardia. This tends to be familial in 30–50% of patients. This is estimated to be the underlying cause of SCD in 20% of those under the age of 35 years.[2]

Bradyarrhythmias can also be an important cause of syncope. Sick sinus syndrome is a good example and can be picked up with history and ECG. Elderly patients with hypothyroidism may present with episodes of syncope with increased background fatigue.

Structural Abnormalities of the Heart

Patients with ischemic heart disease, nonischemic dilated cardiomyopathies, valvular heart disease (both mitral and aortic valve disease), and hypertrophic obstructive cardiomyopathies are prone for syncope. The history of syncope in these situations usually indicates more severe alteration of cardiac hemodynamics. Some of these disorders may have additional arrhythmias and require further cardiac electrophysiological evaluation and decision on implantable defibrillators.

Orthostatic Hypotension

This is similar to vasodepressor neurocardiogenic syncope in the sense that fall in blood pressure is the main abnormality and that the tendency is a more enduring one. Thus, disorders that can cause drop in blood pressure with orthostatic stress are important here. Among the elderly, drug-induced orthostatic hypotension is common, often related to antihypertensive medications and other times related to medicines for prostatism (α-blockers) or Parkinsonism (dopaminergics). History and examination would elicit additional neurological problems beyond autonomic failure. Gait and extrapyramidal dysfunction suggest disorders like multiple system atrophy and peripheral nerve symptoms would suggest inherited or acquired neuropathies with autonomic involvement. Rarely, some patients have pure autonomic failure as a neurodegenerative disorder.

Internal hemorrhage (sudden gastrointestinal bleed or ruptured ectopic pregnancy, ovarian cyst, or rupture of aortic aneurysm) can present with TLOC. There will be systemic (autonomic) features of internal bleeding including hypotension, which can last longer than few minutes. Careful history and examination followed by endoscopy or ultrasound will establish diagnosis.

ALGORITHM

Flowchart 1 gives an algorithm for approach to a patient with TLOC.

SYNCOPE IN GERIATRIC POPULATION

The practice of geriatric medicine involves judgment of contribution of multiple potential contributing factors due to multiple comorbidities. Hence, the causes could be multifactorial related to underlying comorbidities; sometimes the most obvious cause may have the least contribution, medications for the comorbidities could be contributing, and age-related alterations in physiology could increase chances of syncope as well as modify the symptoms during the episode. For example, anterograde amnesia is more common, global hypoperfusion can cause focal symptoms due to preexisting critical cerebral vascular disease, systemic metabolic factors can predispose to syncope, and neurodegenerative disorders with autonomic involvement tend to become more common.

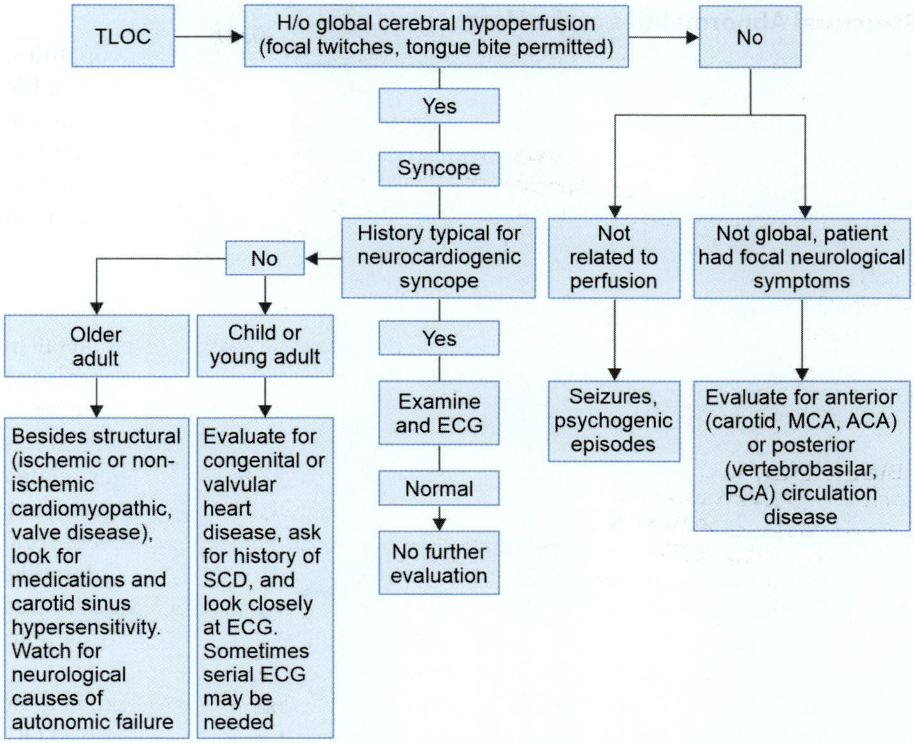

FLOWCHART 1: Algorithm for approaching a patient with transient loss of consciousness.

(ACA: anterior cerebral artery; ECG: electrocardiogram; MCA: middle cerebral artery; PCA: posterior cerebral artery; SCD: sudden cardiac death; TLOC: transient loss of consciousness)

CONCLUSION

Syncope is a TLOC due to GCHP. Presyncope is the term used for symptoms attributed to GCHP short of loss of consciousness or fall. The most common cause for syncope is related to cardiovascular reflexes maintaining blood pressure with change in body position and referred to as neurocardiogenic syncope. Sinister causes for syncope are cardiac, which includes arrhythmias and structural heart disease. Family history of SCD should be specifically asked. Autonomic failure causing orthostatic hypotension will tend to cause more frequent presyncope and intermittent syncope. This is most often related to medications, but can also be a component of central or peripheral neurological disorders. A pathophysiological approach is advocated for differential diagnoses in patients with history of possible syncope.

combinations resulting in temporary failure of blood supply to the cortex. Whereas, in orthostatic hypotension (OH) due to autonomic failure, the reflexes maintaining the cardiovascular integrity are chronically impaired. Cardiogenic syncope may be due to structural cardiac disease or heart-rhythm irregularities, which results in low cardiac output causing cerebral hypoperfusion.[3] The prognosis, underlying pathophysiology, clinical manifestations, and treatment vary among these causes.

TYPES OF SYNCOPE

Neurally Mediated

Vasovagal Syncope

Vasovagal or neurocardiogenic syncope is a type of syncope where the abnormal autonomic function plays the main role. Prolonged standing usually triggers the event, which causes the blood to pool in the legs. Instead of the normal reflex, which includes tachycardia and increase in blood pressure, an abnormal reflex occurs resulting in slow heart rate and relaxed blood vessels, making the blood pressure too low, and thus causing cerebral hypoperfusion.

Reflex Syncope

Reflex syncope is also known as situational syncope where the problem lies in nervous system, which maintains the blood pressure and heart rate with regards to the pain and fear response. It usually results in bradycardia, venous pooling of blood, and low blood pressure, which causes syncope. Sudden withdrawal of normal blood supply to the brain results in transient loss of consciousness. In most of these syncopes, the patients usually regain the consciousness immediately once they lie down, as venous pooling in legs decreases and causes increase in venous inflow to the heart and further rise in cardiac output resulting in normal cerebral perfusion. Some of the triggers for reflex syncope are:

- Coughing
- Eating or swallowing
- Emotional distress including pain and fear
- Prolonged standing
- Defecation
- Micturition

Carotid Sinus Hypersensitivity

In normal individuals, stimulation of carotid sinus causes reflex slowing of sinus rate and atrioventricular conduction. This reflex gets exaggerated in patients with carotid sinus hypersensitivity. This may be due to cardiac conduction slowing, reflex vasodilatation, or a combination of both. The diagnosis is based on the clinical history of reproducibility of similar symptoms with the maneuvers that are known to stimulate the carotid sinus such as shaving, neck massage, or wearing tight collar.[4]

Orthostatic Hypotension

Orthostatic syncope results from an abnormal autonomic nervous system (ANS) response that is provoked by changes in position—particularly prolonged erect posture after being in a supine position for a while. The ANS controls a series of reflexes, which causes heart rate to increase or decrease and regulate the blood pressure when you change position. When a person stands up, the ANS automatically increases the peripheral vascular resistance and causes tachycardia to make sure that enough blood and oxygen get to the brain. If the ANS is not functioning correctly, dizziness or syncope occurs with position changes as in case of:

- Primary autonomic failure—Parkinson's disease, multiple system atrophy, Wernicke's encephalopathy, and multiple sclerosis
- Secondary autonomic failure—spinal cord injury, diabetes, connective tissue disease, and amyloidosis
- Drug-induced—antihypertensives, antianginal, insulin, alcohol, antidepressants, antiparkinsonian agents, etc.
- Volume depletion—vomiting, diarrhea, blood loss, and poor intake.

Cardiac Syncope

Cardiac syncope is characterized by sudden temporary loss of consciousness with momentary premonitory symptoms or without any warning symptoms, which occur due to cerebral hypoperfusion caused by reduction in cardiac output. It can be due to:

- *Abnormal heart rhythm such as:* Sinus node dysfunction, conduction blocks, ventricular tachycardia, supraventricular tachycardia, etc.
- *Abnormal heart structures or blood vessels:* Valvular heart disease, cardiomyopathies, pericardial effusion, coronary artery disease, atrial myxomas, etc.[4]

NEURALLY MEDIATED SYNCOPE

Neurally-mediated syncope refers to all forms of syncope that occur directly from the cardiovascular effects of neural signals originating from the central nervous system and consists of various conditions where the cardiovascular system fails to maintain the arterial blood pressure temporarily in response to certain triggering factors. Normally functioning cardiovascular reflex mechanisms, such as tachycardia and vasospasm, do not occur in these conditions causing reduction in blood pressure and diffuse cerebral hypoperfusion. It consists of vasovagal or neurocardiogenic, carotid hypersensitivity, and reflex or situational syncope.

Reflex syncope is broadly categorized depending on the pathway of reflex mechanisms involved such as afferent or efferent pathways. Efferent pathway disturbances can be again divided into sympathetic or parasympathetic system involvement. Sympathetic dysfunction includes loss of vascular tone in upright posture resulting in hypotension, hence, vasodepressor type. In parasympathetic dysfunction, it causes bradycardia or asystole and is termed cardioinhibitory.

MISCELLANEOUS CAUSES OF SYNCOPE

There are several types of syncope, which cannot be readily classified. More than one mechanism play in these syncopes. Both vasodepressor and cardioinhibitory factors have roles in these but multiple factors are frequent.

Situational Syncope

Situational syncope includes a group of reflex syncopal syndromes that occur in specific circumstances and may have the pathophysiological mechanisms in common or different **(Box 1)**.

The various mechanism involved include:

- Reduction of venous return by increased intrathoracic pressure as in cough syncope
- Sudden reflex peripheral vasodilation due to the release of urinary bladder pressure and slowing of heart rate in micturition syncope
- Excess vasodilation in compensation to environmental heat followed by sudden upright posturing causing sudden volume displacement as getting out from hot tub
- Swallowing cold liquids in overheated state induces esophageal or gastric spasms, which can produce vagal reflex-mediated syncope
- Excruciating pain in outer ear canal leads to increased firing of glossopharyngeal nerve, vagal stimulation, and glossopharyngeal syncope.[10]

Metabolic Disorders-related Syncope

The sudden onset of loss of consciousness depends on onset and reversible nature of the metabolic disturbances. Symptoms are unrelated to posture, but may increase with exercise. Lightheadedness and dizziness are frequent but true syncope rarely occurs. Various causes are hypoxia, hypoglycemia, hyperventilation, electrolyte disturbances such as hypo- or hyperkalemia/calcemia/magnesemia.[11]

Endocrine Disorders-related Syncope

Hypoadrenalism, due to Addison's disease, adrenal suppression, and hypopituitarism, results in OH, and hence, syncope.

Conditions, such as carcinoid syndrome, pheochromocytomas, and mastocytosis, in which substances are produced, which are vasoactive and cause vasodilation, further lead to reduced cardiac output.[10]

BOX 1 Types of situational syncopes.

- Micturition
- Glossopharyngeal
- Deglutition
- Defecation
- Postprandial
- Valsalva
- Sexual activity
- Instrumentation
- Sneeze
- Trumpet playing
- Hot tub
- Cough

Subclavian Steal Phenomenon

Vascular stenosis results in an area of low-pressure distal to the occlusion in the vessel. This results in redirection of blood from a neighboring artery. Subclavian artery stenosis diverts the blood flowing in the ipsilateral vertebral artery distal to the obstruction site causing decline in cerebral blood supply. Syncope occurring during arm exertion should prompt this condition.[12]

Hysterical

Absence of blood pressure and pulse rate and skin color changes or any outward display of anxiety is suggestive of hysterical fainting.[13]

Syncope of Unknown Cause

There are significant proportions of syncope without any identifiable causes, i.e., 33–50% cases as described by Kapoor et al. and 40% in the Framingham Heart Study.[14,15]

CONCLUSION

Syncope is a common presenting symptom and is often a challenging diagnostic dilemma because of its various underlying causes. A careful initial clinical assessment with directed investigation is crucial in arriving at a presumptive diagnosis.

Syncopes, which are neutrally mediated, are characterized by sudden and temporary disturbances in ANS leading to hypotension or bradycardia. The patients with neurocardiogenic syncope have similar outcomes to those who are free of syncope confirming the benign prognosis in these patients. The type of syncope determines the prognosis. Patients and caregivers must be counseled on how to anticipate the syncopal attacks, the dos and don'ts during the episode, how to avoid injuries, and when a hospital transfer would be required. Education and counseling in majority of the patients provide improvement in the avoidance of aggravating factors, adequate hydration, and with medication (when required in some patients).

REFERENCES

1. Jacobsen TN, Morgan BJ, Scherrer U, Vissing SF, Lange RA, Johnson N, et al. Relative contributions of cardiopulmonary and sinoaortic baroreflexes in causing sympathetic activation in the human skeletal muscle circulation during orthostatic stress. Circ Res. 1993;73(2):367-78.
2. Grubb BP, Karas B. Clinical disorders of the autonomic nervous system associated with orthostatic intolerance: An overview of classification, clinical evaluation, and management. Pacing Clin Electrophysiol. 1999;22(5):798-810.
3. Morillo CA, Ellenbogen KA, Fernando Pava L. Pathophysiologic basis for vasodepressor syncope. Cardiol Clinic. 1997;15(2):233-49.
4. Ropper AH, Samuels MA, Klein JP. Adams and Victor's Principles of Neurology, 10th edition. New York: McGraw Hill; 2014. pp. 383-6.

D

E

N

O

P

T

U

V